Challenges in Otorhinolaryngology

Challenges in Otorhinolaryngology

Anil Malhotra
Consultant and Head
Department of ENT
Zulfi General Hospital
Zulfi City
Riyadh Region
Saudi Arabia

Milind Kirtane
Professor of ENT
Seth G.S. Medical College and
KEM Hospital, Mumbai
Consultant ENT Surgeon
PD Hinduja Hospital,
Breach Candy Hospital and
Prince Aly Khan Hospital
Mumbai, India

JAYPEE BROTHERS
MEDICAL PUBLISHERS (P) LTD
New Delhi

Published by

Jitendar P Vij
Jaypee Brothers Medical Publishers (P) Ltd
EMCA House, 23/23B Ansari Road, Daryaganj
New Delhi 110 002, India
Phones: +91-11-23272143, +91-11-23272703, +91-11-23282021,
+91-11-23245672
Fax: +91-11-23276490, +91-11-23245683 e-mail: jpmedpub@del2.vsnl.net.in
Visit our web site: www.jaypeebrothers.com

Branches

- 202 Batavia Chambers, 8 Kumara Krupa Road
  Kumara Park East, **Bangalore** 560 001, Phones: +91-80-22285971,
  +91-80-22382956, +91-80-30614073 Tele Fax : +91-80-22281761
  e-mail: jaypeebc@bgl.vsnl.net.in
- 282 IIIrd Floor, Khaleel Shirazi Estate, Fountain Plaza
  Pantheon Road, **Chennai** 600 008, Phones: +91-44-28262665,
  +91-44-28269897 Fax: +91-44-28262331
  e-mail: jpmedpub@md3.vsnl.net.in
- 4-2-1067/1-3, Ist Floor, Balaji Building, Ramkote Cross Road,
  Hyderabad 500 095, Phones: +91-40-55610020, +91-40-24758498
  Fax: +91-40-24758499 e-mail: jpmedpub@rediffmail.com
- 1A Indian Mirror Street, Wellington Square
  Kolkata 700 013, Phone: +91-33-22451926 Fax: +91-33-22456075
  e-mail: jpbcal@cal.vsnl.net.in
- 106 Amit Industrial Estate, 61 Dr SS Rao Road
  Near MGM Hospital, Parel, **Mumbai** 400 012
  Phones: +91-22-24124863, +91-22-24104532, +91-22-30926896
  Fax: +91-22-24160828 e-mail: jpmedpub@bom7.vsnl.net.in

Challenges in Otorhinolaryngology

First Edition: **2005**

ISBN 81-8061-401-8

Typeset at JPBMP typesetting unit
Printed at Gopsons Papers Ltd, A-14, Sector 60, Noida 201 301, India

List of Contributors

Bartley Jim FRACS
Otolaryngologist,
Green Lane Hospital,
Auckland, New Zealand

D'Cruz Anil K MS, DNB
Consultant, Head and Neck Services
Tata Memorial Hospital
Mumbai, India

Diz Dioz P MD, DDS, PhD
Head of Department,
Special Needs Development,
School of Medicine and Dentistry,
University of Santiago de Compastela, Spain
Vice President, Spanish Society of
Special Needs Dentistry

Garcia Pola M.J. MD DDS PhD
Head of Department,
Oral Medicine, School of Stomatology,
University of Oviedo, Spain.
Founder Member, Spanish
Society of Oral Medicine.

Ignace Wei William

Kacker Santosh K. MS, FRCS, FAMS
Consultant Otorhinolaryngologist.
Ex Director and Professor,
All India Institute of Medical Sciences,
New Delhi, India
Ex President,
Association of Otolaryngologists of India

Kirtane Milind V MS, DORL.
Hon. Prof. of ENT,
Seth GS Medical College and
KEM Hospital, Mumbai.
Consultant ENT Surgeon,
PD Hinduja Hospital, Mumbai, India.
Ex President,
Association of Otolaryngologists of India

Malhotra Anil MS
Consultant and Head
Department of ENT
Zulfi General Hospital
Zulfi City
Riyadh Region
Saudi Arabia

Malhotra N S
ENT Consultant
Guru Nanak Hospital
Mumbai, India

Muranjan Sujata MS DNB, DORL
ENT Consultant
Bombay Hospital
Mumbai, India

Pai Prathamesh S MS, DNB, DORL
Associate Consultant,
Head and Neck Services,
Tata Memorial Hospital,
Mumbai, India

Patel Hetal MS, DNB, DORL
Associate Prof., Dept of ENT,
Seth GS Medical College and
KEM Hospital,
Mumbai, India

Pradhan Sultan A MS, FRCS
Chief, Head and Neck Services,
Tata Memorial Hospital
Mumbai, India

Rao Janardhan J MS, DLO, DNB
Consultant ENT Surgeon,
Apollo Hospitals,
Hyderabad, India

Seoane Leston J MD, DDS, PhD, MPDH
Senior Lecturer Oral Surgery,
Dept. of Stomatology,
School of Medicine and Dentistry,
University of Santiago de Compostela, Spain
Founder Member of Spanish Society of
Oral Medicine; Head of Teaching and
Learning, Regional Army Hospital.

Shah Vinod H MS, DLO, FACS
ENT Surgeon,
Shruti ENT Hospital, Surat, India
Ex President, Association of Otolaryngologists
of India.

Varela Centelles P DDS Med. Sci, MPDH, PhD
Dental Surgeon,
Primary Care Clinics,
Galician Health Service,
Burela (Lugo),
Spain

Yuen APW MS, FRCS, FHKAM, FACS, DLO
Associate Prof. of Otolaryngology,
University of Hong Kong Medical Center,
Queen Mary Hospital,
Hong Kong

Foreword

I have great pleasure having previewed the manuscript of *Challenges in Otorhinolaryngology* and to write a Foreword for it.

Dr Anil Malhotra, who is bringing out his second book at a young age, was an illustrious student of an illustrious teacher, Prof. YN Mehra. I had been hearing about the enormous talents of Anil from various sources and those talents are there for all to see. In 1998, I came across a book *Auditory Evoked Responses in Clinical Practice*, written by Dr Malhotra. I am not an Otoneurologist, but I read the book because the Prologue was written by Prof. Dr SK Kacker and Foreword by Prof. Dr Milind Kirtane. Both of them I know at a personal level as eminent academicians. I found the material fascinating. He has explained in a simplified manner for a beginner like me a vast material for any otoneurologist to read and benefit. During my discussions with various otologists in different parts of the world, the eminent specialists mentioned about this book. The monograph is more read in the western countries of the world than in India.

Prof. Milind Kirtane has been in the forefront, taking the quality of practice of ENT in India to new heights. We have known him, since his early teaching days, as an academician of a high order, having authored chapters in many books, apart from writing his own books. Anil and Milind have combined to form a potent force and we are proud to have such ENT surgeons in the country who are also academicians of the highest order.

In this book, Drs Malhotra and Kirtane have gathered contributors from India and other countries. These include eminent professors and famous academicians from abroad and Indian otorhinolaryngologists who have carved a niche for themselves, including few past Presidents of the Association of Otolaryngologists of India. These authors are known to have done original work in the subject they have contributed. Readers will know the best and the latest on these topics.

There is nothing like the last word in science, but even for the experienced, this material will be the basis for further research. I may mention particularly the Chapters on Vertigo. I found the material enlightening. Meniere described the disease in 1861, but scientists and clinicians still do not have the last word on it because no one dies of Meniere's. The knowledge gained by a Swedish scientist Dr Alexin on the blood supply of the internal ear and the latest imaging techniques, i.e., CT, MRI and PET etc. have clarified many an enigma about vertigo; but one day, hopefully, some other techniques will show what actually occurs during an attack.

The title *Challenges in Otorhinolaryngology* is itself stimulating and thought provoking for the readers. Many of them will follow the authors' lead for further studies to enlarge the horizons of knowledge in the subject. After nearly sixty years of practice in ENT, I still added to my knowledge on various topics discussed. I feel the readers will similarly benefit.

(Padma Bhushan) LH Hiranandani

Preface

A head and neck surgeon has to deal with a wide array of clinical situations in his professional life. Many of them pass off as routine work but some pose a challenge and put his surgical acumen and intellectual skills to a severe test. There are diagnostic tangles to be solved and surgical innovations to be worked up. The examples are many and we decided to take some such challenging situations, understand them and try to propose the best possible solutions. Ostensibly, the leading lights in the business were commissioned to write these chapters. We do not claim that this list of clinical challenges is exhaustive or that there are no better experts in the field than our contributors. We have tried to cover as much distance with as many available experts as possible. It was an honour as well as pleasure to organise so many illustrious authors for contributing to this book, even though it was quite time consuming, given everybody's busy schedules.

We have set in a process and do hope that the endeavour of enlarging the scope of this book will continue with subsequent editions. We will certainly welcome ideas as well as contributions from those of our readers who are credited with expertise in difficult sub-fields of ENT and Head and Neck Surgery. We hope that the present edition will help the practitioners of Otorhinolaryngology as well as groom the fresh postgraduates into learning and achieving more.

We thank our contributors for the hard work they have put into write their chapters. We appreciate the merits of their contents and hope the readers will benefit a lot from them. We are honoured to have the Foreword written by Prof. Dr LH Hiranandani—the grand old man of Indian otolaryngological scene and widely acclaimed as the father of modern otolaryngology in India. His blessings have encouraged us for the present and the future.

Anil Malhotra
Milind Kirtane

Contents

CHAPTER

1

Challenges in Otoplasty

Jim Bartley

Otoplasty loosely means plastic reconstruction or correction of the pinna. A variety of otoplasty techniques have been described. In the current era of "evidence based" medicine, some of these papers belong to the realm of myth and magic. In the real world the choice of technique still remains largely a matter of personal preference; there is postoperative morbidity[1] and complications do occur.[2] A mark of good surgeon is the ability not only to achieve good results but also to both avoid and manage complications. Otoplasty appears a simple operation; in reality care and respect are needed. The neophyte otoplasty surgeon must anticipate a recurrence rate in the order of 10 per cent and use surgical techniques that allow him to salvage the poor result.

The main indications for otoplasty are cosmesis and psychosocial distress.[1] Unlike cartilaginous growth in the nose, auricular cartilage growth is nearly complete by age five.[3] Surgery can be performed before the child starts school without fear of significantly altering ear growth.

Aesthetic Parameters

Aesthetic goals for prominent ear surgery have been described.[4] "Normal" ears are often asymmetrical in their position on the head particularly in their size and degree of protrusion. In most normal ears, especially in the upper third, the helix is visible on front view 2-5 mm laterally behind the antihelix. Helical rims are usually located within 15-20 mm of the scalp. When the helical rims are closer than 10 mm the ears appear "stuck to the head". Asymmetry is less obvious the closer the ears are to the head. While the inter and intraobserver variation in these measurement is probably very high, these measurements are useful intraoperatively to reassure the surgeon that symmetry is being achieved.

Preoperative Consultation

The patient (or the child's parents) must be fully informed preoperatively of the specific goals and limitations of the planned surgery. Asymmetric ears are difficult to make symmetric. Bleeding problems and any tendency to either keloid or hypertrophic scarring needs exclusion. The patient should be specifically warned that there is a possibility that minor revision surgery should be necessary at a later date. Psychiatric evaluation may be necessary in some patients.

Examination

Three aspects need to be assessed:

1. Depth of the conchal bowl
2. The degree of antihelical unfolding
3. The lobule prominence.

Asymmetries in position and size should be noted. The ears should be manipulated medially to assess the cartilaginous consistency, the postauricular skin redundancy and the desired alteration.

Photographic Documentation

Otoplasty involves a considerable learning curve. A surgeon who neglects preoperative and regular postoperative standardised photographic documentation denies himself/ herself a valuable tool for self-education.

Surgical Techniques

The patient's main concern is the degree of prominence. The surgeon's role is to medialise the ear without signs of surgical intervention. The number of techniques described suggests that each has its advantages and disadvantages. The term "otoplasty" denotes simplicity in surgical practice that does not necessarily exist; some ears are more difficult to correct than others and surgery needs to be tailored to the individual ear. The role of the surgical endoscopes in otoplasty has yet to be defined.[5]

Techniques can be grouped into three areas:

1. Antihelical fold creation
2. Conchal bowl reduction
3. Correction of lobular protrusion.

Creation of the Antihelical Fold

The debate first focuses on the relative merits of cartilage cutting versus cartilage sparing procedures in the creation of a normal antihelix. The main advantages of cartilage sparing over cartilage cutting are that the results appear more natural and failures following cartilage-cutting techniques can be very difficult to salvage.

Cartilage scoring was developed by Stenstrom,[6] who showed that disruption of the perichondrium on the anterior surface of the ear cartilage along the proposed antihelix lead to contraction of the intact perichondrium on the posterior side. Posterior scoring, in order to weaken the cartilage to create the antihelical fold, has also been advocated.[7]

Mustardé popularised a technique of cartilage folding by the use of multiple radially placed mattress sutures.[8] These have the advantages of versatility and reversibility. The tension created by mobilising the cartilage is assumed initially by the suture material and subsequently by scar tissue reaction, which forms and splints the cartilage in its new position. Excessive tension on Mustardé sutures may increase the complication rate.[9]

Experimental work creating an antihelical fold with rabbits has shown that results are variable and not necessarily predictable even with the same surgical technique.[10] The same may be true in humans. In children a suture technique or a scoring technique will give adequate results. In adults, a combination of both suture and scoring techniques will be needed to control the inherent spring of mature auricular cartilage. The superior pole in particular has a tendency to lateralise,[9] and should be overcorrected. Experience with a particular technique tailored to the individual ear, rather than a "cook book" procedure, may be the most important factor in achieving a good postoperative outcome.[2]

The Conchal Bowl

If one accepts that any technique of antihelix formation may give variable results even in experienced hands, it is important to reduce the amount of antihelical bending that might be required. Conchal bowl techniques are thus useful adjunctive techniques in otoplasty. A number of techniques are available to reduce the prominence of the conchal bowl. Strips of cartilage may be excised from the lateral aspect of the concha.[11] The beginner surgeon commonly removes too much cartilage in the midportion thus creating a telephone ear. Alternatively, tangential shaving of conchal cartilage, as well as removal of soft tissue, sets the concha back making it less prominent (Fig. 1.1).[12,13] This technique is a particularly safe technique for the occasional surgeon. The concha can also be rotated medially by using concha-mastoid or fossa-triangularis-temporalis fascia sutures. These flatten the concha against the mastoid bone.[14]

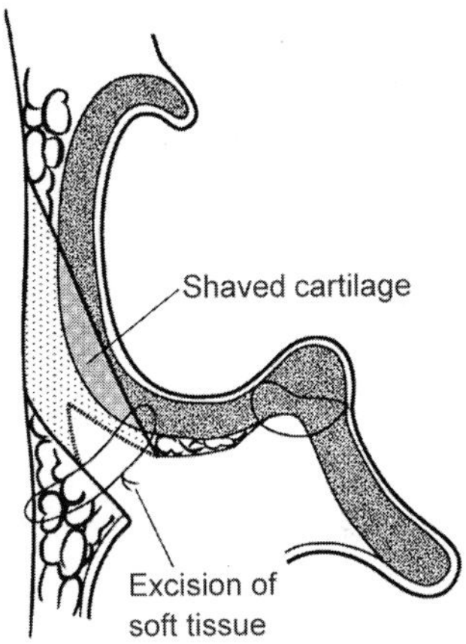

Fig. 1.1: Axial cut through the auricular cartilage showing how shaving of cartilage and soft tissue places the concha medially. Skin is dissected up to the auricular rim. By dissecting skin up to the auricular rim, the pull of the skin is transmitted across the site of the antihelix

The Lobule

Surgery to the lobule is often neglected in otoplasty surgery. Surgical techniques should include division and medial suturing of the cauda helicis. The most reliable way to set back the lobule is to remove skin as well but care needs to be exercised if the lobe is pierced or may be pierced at a later stage.

Personal Technique

Anaesthesia

It is my preference to use general anaesthesia in children or when teaching. Adults can easily be done under local anaesthetic with intravenous sedation. Prophylactic antiemetics are routinely given. The operative procedure starts with the infiltration of Marcaine per cent with 1:80,000 in a supraperichondrial plane posteriorly. The area of posterior skin removal is infiltrated. Local anaesthetic is also injected anteriorly over the site of the proposed new antihelix. After skin preparation individual plastic ear drapes are placed over each ear so that both ears can be visualised during surgery. An alternative is surgical hose with holes cut in the sides.

Skin Incision

An incision is made with a 15-blade knife in the postauricular sulcus starting 0.5cm below the superior attachment of the ear to the scalp. It is continued to just above the lobule. A curving incision is then made over the posterior aspect of the concha approximately 1.5 cm from the rim. An ellipse of skin is then removed leaving the postauricular perichondrium intact. Preservation of a large bed of subcutaneous tissue adjacent to the cartilage facilitates scarring. This helps with the permanent creation of an antihelical fold and the setting back of the concha. Haemostasis is achieved with bipolar cautery.

Conchal Setback

Depending on the degree of protrusion of the walls of the fossa triangularis, cavum and cymba conchae, a variable amount of mastoid soft tissue deep to these three bowls is removed. Dissection is kept 1 cm from the external auditory meatus to reduce the potential for the conchal cartilage to slide forward and stenose the external auditory meatus. The bowls are also reduced in size by tangential shaving of the cartilage (Figs 1.1 and 1.2). The conchal bowl is then sutured to soft tissue over the mastoid.[12,13]

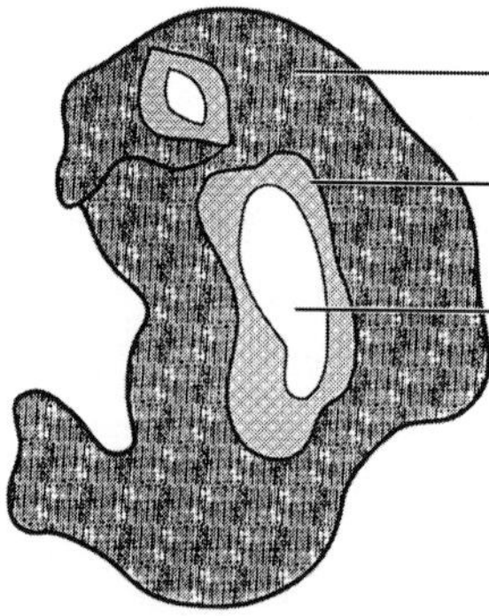

Fig. 1.2: Cartilage is shaved tangentially from the fossa triangularis, cavum and cymbae conchae in order to set back the concha.

Antihelical Fold

Usually, a small incision is made superiorly above the superior crus of the fossa triangularis anteriorly and an anterior tunnel is dissected just lateral to the perichondrium. If identification of the cauda helicis is necessary, this anterior tunnel is dissected starting inferomedial to the cauda helicis. The anterior surface is scored with an otoabrader or toothed forceps until the antihelical fold feels soft and malleable. Posteriorly skin is undermined laterally so that the pull of the skin is transmitted across the site of the new antihelix (Fig. 1.3). External Mustardé Maxon (synthetic clear absorbable monofilament polyglyconate) sutures,[15] are usually used to create the antihelical fold. It is not necessary to mark the site of proposed antihelix. The antihelix is created with finger pressure and the sites of the sutures marked on the lateral side. The suture is then brought out through the skin and cartilage from behind, then placed back though the needle hole, through the skin, back through the needle hole and the cartilage (Fig. 1.4). Further Mustardé sutures are then placed as required (Fig. 1.6).

The Lobule

Contouring of the lobule is achieved by skin removal and suture. When necessary the cauda is freed from the concha.

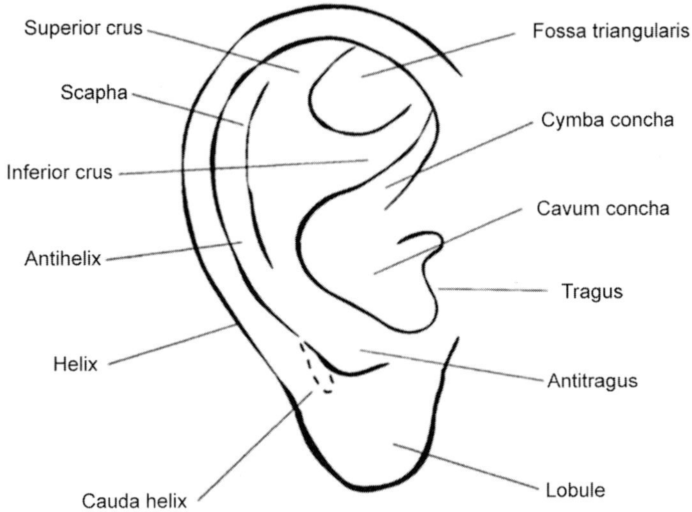

Fig. 1.3: External ear anatomy

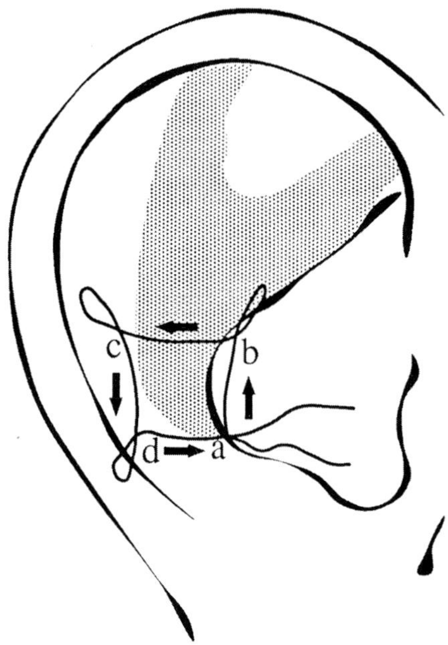

Fig. 1.4: The needle is placed through the cartilage from behind the ear to exit the anterior surface at the marked spot "a". The needle hole is then used to feed the suture under the skin to the marked spot "b". At "b" the needle is again placed through the suture exit hole to pierce the cartilage and appear posteriorly. The needle is placed through the cartilage from behind the ear to exit at the marked spot "c". The needle how is then used to feed the suture under the skin to the marked spot "d". At "d" the needle is again placed through the suture hole to pierce the cartilage to appear posteriorly. The suture is then slowly tightened and the resulting antihelical fold examined. When the fold appears adequate further throws are then placed to hold the antihelical fold in place

Closure and Bandaging

Skin closure is effected with a continuous subcutaneous 4.0 Vicryl in younger children; a continuous 4.0 Nylon is used in older children. Following closure of the second ear attention is made to symmetry. If ears are asymmetrical in position or prominence one ear can be readjusted using sutures. Tulle gras dressing is placed in the conchal bowl and scapha. A dressing is placed in the postauricular sulcus and a firm head dressing applied. This is removed the following 24-48 hours later. There is no need for patients to have head bandaging for 7-10 days postoperatively.[16] The patient is then advised to wear a cotton headband at night for six weeks.

Postoperative Care

The only prospective study of postoperative morbidity reported significant problems with bandage displacement, pain, vomiting and itch in children. Unless specifically asked for these problems are not usually reported back to the surgeon.[1] If a subcuticular Nylon stitch was used it is removed at seven days.

Early Complications

Haematoma

If overnight bleeding occurs from behind the wound a further pressure dressing is placed. If a haematoma occurs it is relatively easily evacuated under general anaesthetic the following day and a further head dressing applied for 24 hours.

Infection

Infection is extremely rare and can result in cellulitis and perichondritis following otoplasty. Staphylococcus, *E. coli* and Pseudomonas have been reported.

Late Complications

Suture Complication

Permanent sutures if not white may be seen through the skin. A high incidence of granuloma formation (up to 8per cent) is reported,[9] when permanent sutures are used to reconstruct the antihelix. If granulomas do occur the granuloma and the precipitating sutures can usually be removed several months later without any loss of correction.

Hypertrophic and Keloid Scars

This complication is rare but does occur. Keloid, in my experience, occurs 9-18 months after the original surgery. In my opinion, excessive wound tension is a major factor and one should evaluate one's surgical technique. Keloid scars should settle with excision of the scar and steroid injection but limited radiotherapy may be necessary.

Poor Result

Dissatisfied Patient

Postoperative satisfaction does not correlate with the quality of the repair. There may be a small group of patients who may be dissatisfied despite an adequate result.[1]

Telephone Ear Deformity

Telephone ear deformity is the result of overly enthusiastic correction of the middle third segment of the ear. This deformity may follow excessive removal of postauricular skin, mastoid soft tissue or conchal cartilage. It can be difficult to salvage.

Recurrence

Loss of correction with recurrence will in general be evident by 3 months after surgery. Messner and Crysdale have reported a recurrence rate of 33 per cent.[17] Unwinding of the superior pole is commonly seen in clinical practice. Common cause of surgical failure is—

1. Improper placement of insufficient number of sutures. When using a Mustardé suture technique careful attention needs to be given to the superior pole.
2. Cartilage to strong to be controlled with sutures
3. Insufficient scoring to weaken the cartilage
4. Failure to anticipate unwinding of the superior pole.

Occasional surgeons must anticipate a recurrence rate of at least 10 per cent regardless of the technique used. The most common cause, in my experience, is insufficient weakening particularly at the superior pole.

Overcorrected Ear

Techniques correcting the over corrected ear have been described.[18] Although not ideal most patients are happy if their ears are overcorrected.

Obliteration of the Postauricular Sulcus

If skin is removed over the mastoid surface the potential for loss of the sulcus exists. Techniques correcting this have been described although long-term results are not reported.[18]

Antihelical Deformities

Cartilage cutting techniques require more aggressive surgery and have a greater risk for causing sharp ridges or irregular contours along the new antihelix. Although the results may be excellent in the immediate postoperative period anterior surface irregularities slowly become apparent within 6-12 months. Anterior cartilage scoring and rasping rarely cause a roughened irregular surface.

Ear Lobe Deformities

Ear lobe protrusion is common but again usually not of concern to the patient.

Results

The evidence suggests that the complication and morbidity rate is higher than many surgeons care to admit. Most reports are based on small, personal, incomplete, retrospective surveys; no large prospective audit of otoplasty has yet been published. The beginner will have initial problems with recurrence in the upper pole; if a cartilage sparing technique is used then the result can be easily retrieved under local anaesthetic in the office.

Conclusions

Most otoplasty papers belong to the realm of myth and magic. Surgeons only show their good results and discuss technique variations. In the real world a learning curve exists, postoperative morbidity occurs[1] and complications are common.[2] With conservative, safe techniques these problems can be addressed. Fortunately patients are less critical than surgeons and are usually extremely grateful after surgery (Figs 1.5a and b and 1.6a and b).

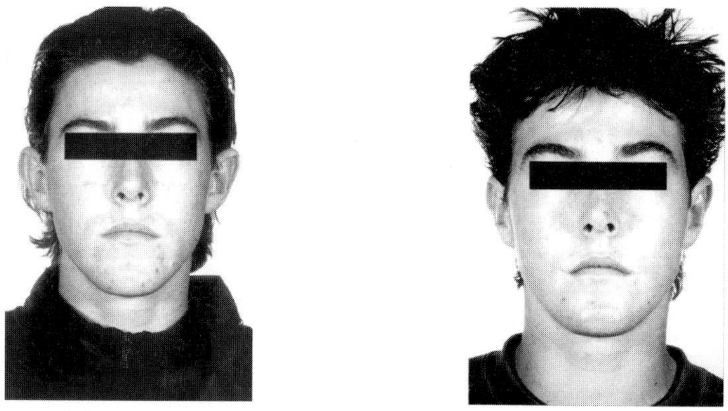

A B

Fig. 1.5a: Preoperative photograph of a 15-year-old male with prominent ears
Fig. 1.5b: Postoperative result at 4 months using only conchal setback

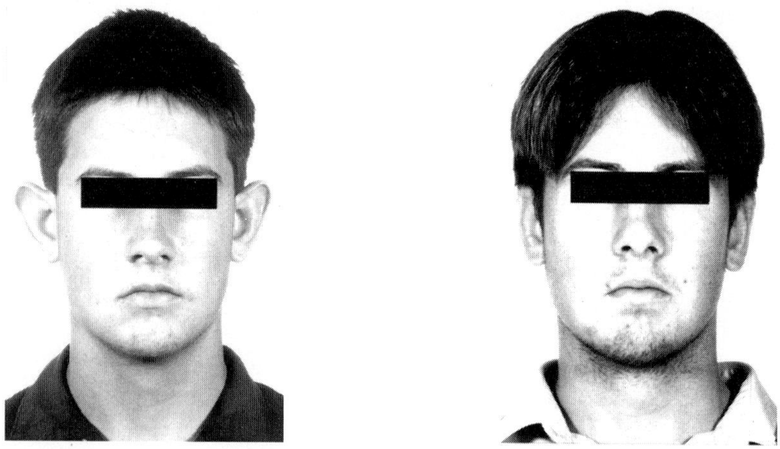

A B

Fig. 1.6a: Preoperative photograph of a 16-year-old male with prominent ears
Fig. 1.6b: Postoperative result at 8 months. A new antihelical fold has been created and the concha setback

Further Viewing

Webster RC (1977) Otoplasty Parts I and II Video. American Academy of Facial Plastic and Reconstructive Surgery.

REFERENCES

1. Bradbury ET, Hewison J, Timmons MJ. Psychological and social outcome of prominent ear correction in children. Br J Plast Surg 1992; 45: 97-100.
2. Calder JC, Naasan A. Morbidity of otoplasty a review of 562 consecutive cases. Br J Plast Surg 1994; 47: 170-74.
3. Adamson JE, Horton CE, Crawford HH. The growth pattern of the external ear. Plast Reconstr Surg 1965; 36: 466-70.
4. McDowell AJ. Goals in otoplasty for protruding ears. Plast Reconstr Surg 1968; 41: 17- 21.
5. Hagerty TA, Barone EJ, Cohen IK. Endoscopic otoplasty in the rabbit model: Effect of mechanical abrasion on the ear cartilage deformation. Plast Reconstr Surg 1998; 101: 487-93.
6. Stenstrom SJ. A natural technique for correction of congenitally prominent ears. Plast Reconstr Surg 1963; 32: 283-93.
7. Pilz S, Hintringer T, Bauer M. Otoplasty using a spherical metal head dermabrader to form a retroauricular furrow: Five year results. Aesth Plast Surg 1995; 19: 83-91.
8. Mustardé JC. The correction of prominent ears by using simple mattress sutures. Br J Plast Surg 1963; 16: 170-78.
9. Adamson PA, McGraw BL, Tropper GJ. Otoplasty: Critical review of clinical results. Laryngoscope 1991; 101: 883-88.
10. Rohrich RJ, Freidman RM, Liland DL. Comparison of otoplasty techniques in the animal model. Ann Plast Surg 1995; 34; 43-47.
11. Stucker FJ, Christiansen TA. The lateral conchal resection technique. Laryngoscope 1977; 87: 58-62.
12. Wright WK. Basic science approach to otoplasty for prominent ears. Otolaryngology 1978; 86: 197-200.
13. Bartley J. Conchal setback in otoplasty. Aust J Otolaryngol 1997; 2: 605-08.
14. Furnas DW. Correction of prominent ears by concha-mastoid sutures. Plast Reconstr Surg 1968; 42: 189-93.
15. Connolly A, Bartley J. "External" Mustardé suture and otoplasty. Clin Otolaryngol 1998; 23: 97-9.
16. Bartley J. How long should ears be bandaged after otoplasty. J Laryngol Otol 1998; 112: 431-32.
17. Messner AM, Crysdale WS. Otoplasty: Clinical protocol and long term results. Arch Otolaryngol Head Neck Surg 1996; 122: 773-77.
18. Walter C, Klein K. Cartilage incision and excision technique. Facial Plastic Surg 1994; 10: 277-86.

CHAPTER 2

Vertigo—An Overview

Anil Malhotra

Consider the following situations:

1. A middle-aged man gets up from his bed in the morning, feels the world spinning around him, holds on to his bed for a minute and then feels better.
2. A middle-aged woman complains to her doctor that again and again, at intervals of two or three months, she gets episodes of giddiness, buzzing sounds in her ears and is progressively getting deafer.
3. A young man, while getting wax curetted out from his ear, feels a very bad sensation of black out and faints.
4. An old woman, climbing stairs slowly, simply drops down.

These are common occurrences in our day-to-day life. On the surface, these appear similar and are loosely called 'dizziness'. This general term encompasses in its ambit various sensations like floating, disorientation, the surroundings rotating, a feeling of being pushed forwards, a blackout, lightheadedness or just being out of touch with reality.

Not all of them are true 'vertigo', which derives its nomenclature from a latin word 'vertere' that means 'to turn around'. The Webster dictionary defines vertigo as 'a disturbance in which the external world seems to revolve around the individual or in which the individual seems to revolve in space'. Cawthorne[1] defined it as 'a hallucination of movement, ….., can be applied to any movement, provided that it does not exist outside the senses of the sufferer'. For diagnostic and therapeutic purposes, as we shall see later, it is important to make a distinction between true vertigo, which is a balance disorder, from other dizzy sensations.

Vertigo is an illusion of rotation or tilting or, uncommonly, being thrown forwards and relates to disturbances in the peripheral or central vestibular system. Vasovagal attacks and hypotensive episodes are faints or near faints giving light headed, blackout sensation and are due to decreased oxygen supply to brain due to causes like orthostatic hypotension, vasovagal stimulation, cardiac arrhythmia, hyperventilation, etc. A very wretched, out of the body sensation is felt in panic disorders while hypoglycaemia gives rise to a confused, light headed and disoriented feeling.

Figures about incidence of vertigo vary but it is generally believed that it accounts for nearly one out of twenty consultations in general practice. In a study from a general medical OPD,[2] dizziness was the third most frequent complaint of the patients.

Till a few decades back, there was helplessness even among experts, while diagnosing and treating many disequilibrium disorders. According to Terence Cawthorne, arguably the father of modern labyrinthology,[1] "The overwhelming vertigo, the awful sickness, and the turbulent eye movements – all enhanced by the slightest movement of the head—combine to form a picture of helpless misery that has few parallels in the whole field of injury and disease". The British Medical Journal[3] quoted, in 1969, WB Mathews, a well known neurologist of those times, "There can be few physicians, so dedicated to their art, that they do not experience a slight decline in their spirits on learning that their patient's complaint is giddiness". LBW Jonkees, one of the pioneers of advanced electronystagmography, opined in 1978, that about 50 per cent of these cases were not solved even with a multidisciplinary approach of connoisseurs in the field.

Not any more though, as we shall see in this and the three succeeding chapters, owing to the rapid strides made in understanding the disease process in our vestibular system.

SOME BASIC CONSIDERATIONS

The ability of normal people to maintain balance and to orient themselves in space comes from three sensors—the eyes, the vestibular apparatus and the proprioceptors. The first information about orientation comes from the eyes, which tell where and in what form the body is situated at a given point of time.

The inner ear consists of cochlear labyrinth and the vestibular labyrinth. The vestibular labyrinth, responsible for equilibrium maintenance, has three semicircular canals and an otolith organ. The semicircular canals are situated in roughly the horizontal, coronal and sagittal planes. The otolith organ consists of utricle and saccule. The apparatus is filled with a fluid called endolymph and each part contains a moveable wedge-like, gelatinous structure called cupula, which carries a large number of large sensitive hairs. It is the movement of endolymph, which bends these hairs and causes impulses to generate regarding body movement. The semicircular canals generate information about angular or rotatory movement, while utricle and saccule sense linear movement.

The VIII cranial nerve connects this vestibular apparatus to the brainstem which has four vestibular nuclei – the medial nucleus, which is the principle and the largest one; the descending or spinal nucleus, the superior nucleus and the lateral nucleus. These nuclei make connections with the nuclei of the III, IV and VI cranial nerves through the medial longitudinal bundle; with the cerebellum through the vestibulo-cerebellar tract and with the spine through the descending portion of medial longitudinal bundle and the vestibulo-spinal tract.

Tonic impulses are being constantly generated from the right and left vestibular labyrinth, from the eyes and from proprioceptors located in muscles, joints neck and in the eyeballs (ocular proprioceptors). These impulses converge at the brainstem and are then led to cortex, which compares the various inputs and integrates them to give an overall assessment of body position at any given moment. In response to this, messages flow from the cortex for maintaining muscle tone and to trigger corrective muscular actions to maintain stable body position. When a person is looking straight and neck is not turned, these impulses are in harmony. The right and left vestibular tonic impulses cancel out each other and a sense of balance and rest is felt.

When the head is rotated to, say left, the movement of endolymph in the right (outer) ear vestibule is faster and that in the left (inner) ear is slower. So a much more brisker generation of impulses on the right, and less on the left, is interpreted by the brain as head turning to left.

If, on the other hand, the left ear vestibular labyrinth is diseased, there is a poor generation of impulses on the left and much brisker messages from the right labyrinth, the brain interprets it much the same way as head rotating towards left. This is vertigo. Rapid head movements will worsen vertigo because they accentuate any imbalance within the vestibular system.

Likewise, if any part of the integrated impulses (vestibular, visual and proprioceptive) gives a contradictory input, the integration gets into utter confusion and leads to vertigo. Roller-coaster ride or even its simulation leads to vertigo due to mismatch between vestibular, visual and proprioceptive inputs. Sometimes, as we shall see in case of the elderly group, many more deficits can summate to produce disability.

If the utricle and saccule are damaged on one side (uncommonly), impulses from the healthy side give an illusory sensation of linear movement.[4]

If the vestibular damage is bilateral and symmetrical, as may happen in ototoxicity, then no vertigo will result because generation (or nongeneration) of impulses on both sides is symmetrical and balanced.

Usually, over a period of time, the brain learns to suppress the over stimulation activity from one side. This is called adaptation or compensation and can be accelerated by some exercises. Indeed, in some cases, the damaged labyrinth may itself develop a capability of sending its own information. Thus, there is hardly any vertigo due to vestibular damage in a vestibular schwannoma, since it is a very slow growing tumour and gives ample time for adaptation. However, even after compensation has occurred, head movements or change in posture may still trigger vertigo for some more time.

If eye proprioception (position or direction of eyeball within the orbit) and neck proprioception (neck turning) do not match, it gives rise to visual vertigo.[5] It occurs in patients with high visual field dependence, who have additional central nervous system symptoms or squint symptoms that lead to inappropriate postural reactions in the face of conflicting sensory symptoms.

Apart from vertigo, the patient may also exhibit autonomic symptoms like sweating, pallor slow thready pulse, nausea and vomiting. This is due to adverse influence of pathological vestibular impulses on the adjoining and interconnecting pathways like that of the vagus nerve.

NYSTAGMUS

It is a rhythmic oscillation of the eyeballs and can be produced physiologically too, while optimising visual orientation during head movements. Pathologically, it is produced when an altered input passes from the vestibular nuclei to the nuclei of III, IV and VI nerves through the medial longitudinal bundle and related pathways in the reticular formation. It may be produced by peripheral (vestibular labyrinthine) or central (brainstem, cerebellar) pathologies and broadly speaking, is horizontal or vertical. Horizontal nystagmus has two components – fast and slow. The slow component is the one actually caused by the pathology, whereas fast component is a corrective effort which brings the eyeball quickly back to original position.

If the nystagmus is elicited by turning the head in the direction of the fast component, it is I degree nystagmus. If the nystagmus can be elicited by looking straight, it is II degree nystagmus. Going a step further, if the nystagmus can be elicited in the above two states plus also when the head is turned in a direction of the slow component, it is III degree nystagmus.

AETIOLOGY OF VERTIGO

The causes of vertigo can be found in the peripheral vestibular apparatus, the central vestibular system, the proprioceptors, and the eyes and may be tabulated in the following manner:

A. Peripheral Causes

I. *Tympanogenic Disease*

1. *Perilymphatic fistula*
   i. Congenital dehiscences
   ii. Spontaneous – sneezing, coughing, raised intracranial tension
   iii. External trauma
   iv. Surgical trauma
   v. Cholesteatomatous erosion
   vi. Infective erosion
   vii. Neoplastic erosion
2. *Inflammatory disease*
   i. Serous otitis media
   ii. Suppurative otitis media

II. *Labyrinthogenic Disease*

1. Congenital malformations and syndromes
2. Traumatic
   a. Fracture of temporal bone
   b. Labyrinthine concussion
3. Traumatic – degenerative
   Benign Paroxysmal Positional Vertigo
4. Inflammatory
   a. Acute
      i. Viral labyrinthitis
      ii. Bacterial labyrinthitis
         Diffuse
         Circumscribed
   b. Chronic
      Tubercular labyrinthopathy
      Syphilitic labyrinthopathy
5. Vascular
   a. Anemia
   b. Hyperviscocity syndrome
   c. Arteriosclerotic labyrinthopathy
   d. Internal auditory artery thrombosis
   e. Leukaemic labyrinthopathy
   f. Haemorrhage in the labyrinth
   g. Hypertensive labyrinthopathy
6. Neoplastic
   a. Invasive – Carcinoma, sarcoma, lymphoma
   b. Erosive – Glomus tympanicum
7. Metabolic and degenerative
   a. Labyrinthine otosclerosis
   b. Paget's disease

c. Drug toxicity
  i. Ototoxic drugs
  ii. Hypoglycaemic drugs
  iii. Psychotropic drugs

8. Miscellaneous
   Endolymphatic hydrops
   Ménière's disease
   Syphilis
   Autoimmune disorder of labyrinth

B. Central Disorders

1. Congenital malformations, cysts and tumours
2. Traumatic – concussion
   i. Cerebellar
   ii. Cerebral
3. Inflammatory
   a. Basal meningitis
   b. Encephalitis
   c. Brain abscess
4. Space occupying lesions
   a. Neoplasms
      i. Hemispheric
      ii. Cerebellopontine angle tumours
      iii. Secondaries
      iv. Lymphoma
      v. Intramural tumours
   b. Arachnoid cyst
   c. Granulomas
5. Vascular
   a. Apoplexy
   b. Transient ischaemic attacks in vertebrobasilar complex
   c. Chronic vertebrobasilar insufficiency
   d. Subclavian Steal syndrome
   e. Wallenberg syndrome
   f. Basilar migraine
   g. Anterior inferior cerebellar artery syndrome
   h. Posterior inferior cerebellar artery syndrome
   i. AV malformation in vertebrobasilar system
   j. Arteriosclerotic disease in vertebrobasilar system
6. Demyelination / Degeneration
   a. Multiple sclerosis
   b. Spinocerebellar degeneration and other degenerative diseases
   c. Dementia
7. Sensory (vertiginous) epilepsy.

C. Mixed/Miscellaneous Origin

1. Psychogenic vertigo
   a. Neurosis
   b. Psychosis
2. Vertigo of old age
3. Motion sickness
4. Ocular vertigo
5. Cervical vertigo

However, only a few among these causes are commonly seen.

Distinction between Peripheral and Central Vertigo

Vertigo can result from lesions in such diverse locations as the vestibular labyrinth, deep paravertebral stretch receptors of the neck, visual/ vestibular interaction centres in the brainstem and cerebellum and in the subjective sensation pathways of thalamus and cortex. It is necessary to diagnose, from management point of view, the peripheral or central origin of vertigo. One can distinguish between the two in the following ways.

1. Vertigo resulting from labyrinthine lesions may be associated with otological and clinical features like deafness, tinnitus, ear discharge, etc. whereas vertigo of central origin is always accompanied by neurological deficits like diplopia, dysarthria, motor/ sensory deficits, even though these may sometimes be of transient nature, as in vertebrobasilar insufficiency. Vertigo originating from C.P. angle lesions may be associated with facial paralysis or numbness and cerebellar ataxia.
2. Vertigo of peripheral origin tends to have abrupt onset and, with central compensation, fades off in a few weeks. Vertigo of Ménière's disease is recurrent. On the other hand, vertigo of central origin tends to develop gradually. But once developed, sustains.
3. Peripheral vestibular lesions impair balance but the patient can still walk during the acute phase. Patients with central lesions cannot stand or take a step without falling.[6]
4. Nausea and vomiting is severe at the onset of vertigo in peripheral lesions but is not so severe in central pathologies.
5. While it is possible to lose consciousness in central lesions, that does not happen in labyrinthine lesions.
6. Spontaneous nystagmus occurs in both the conditions but nystagmus of peripheral origin is prominent only for first 12–24 hours, and in a few days, may be completely inhibited whereas the central nystagmus stays for months.
7. The nystagmus caused by peripheral lesions can be inhibited with fixation. Not so in central type.
8. In peripheral lesions, the nystagmus accentuates on looking towards the fast phase and diminishes on looking towards the slow phase. In central lesions, it will accentuate on either side, i.e. it changes directions.
9. The severity of nystagmus is proportionate to that of vertigo in peripheral lesions. Not so in central lesions.
10. While the nystagmus is horizontal or pendular in the peripheral type, it can be anything—horizontal, oblique, rotatory or tortional in the central variety.

11. While there is a latency of about 10–20 seconds in peripheral type, there is no latency in central.
12. Nystagmus of peripheral type is fatigable.

It may be remembered that infarction of inferior cerebellum may mimic labyrinthine lesions.[7]

VERTIGO IN OLD AGE

With the expectancy of life gradually increasing, there are more old people on earth than before. Vertigo is seen to be a particularly common problem among the elderly. A study[8] of 500 elderly patients over 65 years of age in the English industrial city of Sheffield found that almost half of the men and more than half of the women complained of vertiginous symptoms.

It is quite safe to assume that with the whole body ageing after a certain age, the labyrinth must also age. It has indeed been found[9] that the labyrinth becomes more active in the middle age up to the early sixties and thereafter its activity declines. It was also noted in the same study that although increasing giddiness and deafness were both generally regarded as ageing effects, they do not follow the same pattern.

And what about the central vestibular system? From the 100 ml of blood that a child's brain receives every minute, for every 100 gm of brain tissue, the figure falls to only 50 ml in the adult and to 35 ml in the healthy elderly individual. In old people with symptomatic cerebrovascular disease, the figure must be even lower. Add to it the decrease in the ability of red blood cells to bind oxygen. Superimposed on this are occasions when the vessels become momentarily blocked because neck or body movements put pressure on them.

Fatty deposits have been seen in innumerable autopsies to affect the carotid arteries, the vertebrals and the intracranial arteries. Consider an atherosclerotic vertebral artery along with cervical spondylitis or rheumatoid spondylitis. When such a person raises his/her hand or suddenly turns the head, it causes momentary fall in vertebrobasilar perfusion pressure resulting in a transient ischaemic attack.

The problem in old age does not stop there. The neurons in brain start degenerating. The effects of decreased cerebrovascular perfusion are sudden and focal whereas the effects of neuronal degeneration are slow and diffuse. In various series of autopsies, where the brains of elderly people were examined,[10] less than 10 per cent showed evidence of vascular changes whereas more than half had atrophy of neurons.

There are still more handicaps. The other cogs in the wheel, the eyes and the proprioceptors, are also jeopardised. There are senile changes in the eyes. The muscle tone is generally weak. The response messages from the cortex do not produce a brisk corrective balance. Old people are generally wary of going out alone. They fear a fall. Dizziness is not the only cause of their falls. Old people generally fall on the roads or from the stairs. Ascending the stairs is more hazardous as the old man has to tilt the neck up. If perchance, the old man is suffering from Benign Paroxysmal Positional Vertigo ('the top of the shelf vertigo', more common in old age), he is liable to fall backwards. Vasovagal attacks, arrhythmias, use of hypotensive drugs; orthostatic hypotension and idiopathic syncope[11] are some of the chief causes why old people fall. Once they fall, they are more prone to suffer major trauma as compared to younger population.[12]

Old people, especially women, are more prone to have 'drop attacks', where the victim suddenly, without warning and usually without getting giddy or unconscious, simply falls. The cause is not clear-probably a severe loss of muscle tone in the legs or a petit mal seizure.

PSYCHOGENIC VERTIGO

Psychiatric problems and giddiness have a two-way traffic between them. In a study,[13] about 9 per cent dizzy patients were found to have a psychogenic origin of the complaint. Yet another study[14] reported panic attacks, anxiety states and depression due to vertigo and concluded that psychological sequelae were common in vestibular disorders.

Sigmund Freud believed that giddiness in anxious persons was due to deep-seated emotional conflicts. Psychiatrists tend to agree that vertigo results from dammed up tensions within the patient's mind. These conflicts are unknown to the patient. Once they are brought in to consciousness, they cease to cause symptoms. For diagnosing a psychogenic vertigo, the following criteria must be adhered to:

1. Absence of any demonstrable organic disease.
2. Vague nature of sufferer's complaint.
3. Highly dramatic way in which the patient describes the symptoms.
4. Presence of emotional stress.

There is a lot of debate regarding the relation of psychosis, especially schizophrenia with vertigo but it is beyond the scope of this chapter to go in to those finer details.

MOTION SICKNESS

Humankind has known a feeling of sickness, when using a passive transport, from times immemorial. It ranges from seasickness to journey in the hills. Subjects might become sick when being on a bus, a car, a spacecraft or an airplane for the first time at least. The term 'nausea' is derived from the Greek 'naus', meaning 'ship'. Motion sickness is commonly associated with nausea, retching, vomiting, pallor and perspiration. Since most of these symptoms depict imbalance of autonomic nervous system, one is tempted to regard this process as autonomic disturbance. But this notion has been dispelled by one simple observation. To have motion sickness, one must have an intact vestibular system, even though vestibular information received by brain in itself is not enough to produce sickness. Motion sickness is also felt in simulated states, when the subject is still but some objects undergoing rapid acceleration or rotation are being screened in front of him.

So it all boils down to the fact that motion sickness is the result of conflicting information about the body's position and orientation, coming from various sources like eyes, vestibular system and the proprioceptors. It happens when brain mal-adapts to the information it receives from these sources in contrast to its own stored information. Motion sickness abates when the body gets a chance and time to adapt.

TREATMENT STRATEGIES

The overview makes it quite clear that unless there are clear focal features pointing to a particular area, there is need to investigate the peripheral vestibular system, the central nervous system and the cardiovascular system. A good history, taken painstakingly, can clinch the diagnosis.

The treatment of vertigo may be divided into three parts—specific, symptomatic and rehabilitative.

Specific treatment is the treatment of the cause itself.

Symptomatic treatment involves suppressing the vertigo and taking care of other attendant clinical features. When the vertigo is acute, there may be prostration, vomiting and dehydration. In such a situation, the patient is to be given vestibular suppressants like meclizine, cinnarizine, dimenhydrinate, promethazine, diazepam; antiemetics like prochlorperazine and metoclopramide by parenteral route, along with supportive measures like IV fluids. Once the acuteness subsides, these drugs are to be taken off because they cause sedation, which is a big hindrance in compensation process. If an antivertiginous drug is needed, a non-sedating one like Betahistine Hydrochloride should be used. The thrust of long-term treatment is on rehabilitation that involves vestibular habituation exercises. These exercises quicken adaptation.

REFERENCES

1. Cawthorne T. Vestibular injuries. Proc R Soc Med, 1945; 39:270.
2. Kroenke K, Mangelsdorff AD. Common symptoms in ambulatory care: Incidence, evaluation, therapy and outcome. Am J Med, 1989; 86:262-66.
3. Br Med J, (1969)1:457.
4. Daroff RB. Am Fam Physician 1977; 16:143.
5. Black FO; Vestibular changes in vertigo; Geriatrics 1975; 30:123.
6. Curry JN and Mastuo V. The use of clonazepam in the treatment of nystagmus and related oscillopsia. Ophthalmology 1986; 93: 924-32.
7. Baloh RW. The Lancet 1998; 352: 1841-46.
8. Narrving B, Magnusson M, Holtas S. Isolated acute vertigo in the elderly; vestibular or vascular disease? Acta Neurol. Scand 1995; 91:4348.
9. Droller H and Pembertom J. Vertigo in a random sample of elderly people living in their homes. J. Laryngol. Otol.; 1953; 67:689.
10. Bruner A and Norris TW. Age related changes in caloric nystagmus. Acta Otolaryngol. Suppl: 1971; 282.
11. Wells CE. The role of stroke in dementia. Stroke 1978; 9:1.
12. Foote DO. Prospective evaluation of unexplained syncope, dizziness and falls among community dwelling elderly adults J Gerontol; 1998; 53A: M435-40.
13. Kapoor WN, Snustad D, Peterson J et al. Am J Med 1986; 80:410–28.
14. Drachman DA and Hart CW. An approach to the dizzy patient; Neurology 1972; 22:323.

CHAPTER 3

Benign Paroxysmal Positional Vertigo

SK Kacker

One Mr ML, 50-year-old patient, presented to us with the history of acute attacks of vertigo, which were precipitated when he accidentally turned to left side when lying down. The attack of dizziness would start a few seconds after the assumption of offending position. It would last for approximately one minute and was associated with feeling of nausea and dizziness. On repeatedly assuming the same offending position, the vertigo became less marked and nausea was reduced. He had no loss of consciousness or any weakness of limbs during the attacks. There was no loss of hearing or fullness of ears complained of by the patient during the attacks. The detailed examination and investigations revealed no gross systemic or local disease. The rotatory tests, caloric test audiological studies and CAT scans of brain and ears were normal. The positional tests were positive.

The patients who get such vertigo attacks in the offending position of head without any other positive finding are diagnosed to be suffering from benign paroxysmal positional vertigo[1,4,14] (Barany, 1921, Dix and Hallpike, 1952, Nylen, 1931).

AETIOLOGY

The benign paroxysmal positional vertigo (BPPV) is a symptom complex seen in a variety of conditions, i.e. head injury, vascular lesion, otologic surgery, acute and chronic inflammatory diseases of ear and ageing.

Head Injury

BPPV is a common complaint in cases of head injury. It is found to be present in 47% of patients with longitudinal fracture of the temporal bone and in 20.8% cases of head injury of same severity but no fracture of the temporal bone[3] (Barber,1964). About 24% of patients of Harrison and Ozsahinoglu[10] (1972) complaining of positional vertigo had a previous history of head injury. Head injury causes dislodgement of otoconia from utricular maculae. These dislodged particles migrate to posterior semicircular canal (PSC) (Fig. 3.1).

Vascular Lesion

Barber,1975[2], reported vertebrobasilar deficiency as a common cause of vertigo in patients of middle age and elderly. Typical positional vertigo may be seen in some of the cases. This

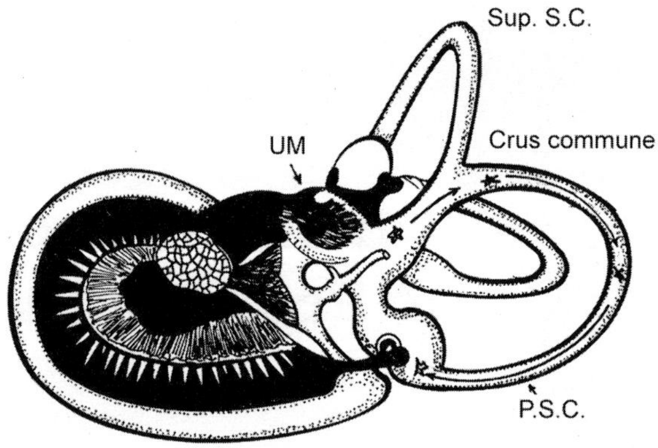

Fig. 3.1: Showing the path taken by otoconia to posterior semicircular canal (PSC.)

problem could be due to degenerative changes in the otoconia causing particles of calcium rich material to be dislodged and migrate to the posterior semicircular canal.

Otologic Surgery

Otologic surgery can lead to delayed degenerative changes and precipitate BPPV. In cases of otosclerosis positional vertigo has been seen. Morales-Garcia and Goycoolea,[12] (1997) have quoted Morales-Garcia (1972)[13] as having reported electronystagmographic abnormalities including positional nystagmus in cases of otosclerosis. Acute and chronic inflammatory diseases of ear may be associated with BPPV (Gacek, 1987).[8]

Idiopathic

In a number of cases, no cause may be detected. Such cases are called idiopathic. Their prognosis is good if no lesion is detected on investigations.

PATHOPHYSIOLOGY

Pathophysiology of the BPPV is due to ampullary dysfunction secondary to the loose pieces of otoconia floating freely in the endolymph and/or found attached to cupula of the posterior semicircular canal.

The semicircular canals—superior, posterior and lateral—three on each side, have a dilated end, which is called ampullary end. The semicircular canals open in the vestibule with two openings—a common opening called crus commune for superior and posterior canals and a separate opening for lateral canals.

The ampullary end of the canals contains a saddle-shaped ridge called crista. The sensory cells of the vestibular epithelium are collected in it. In each ampulla, a gelatinous, wedge-shaped cupola sits astride the crista. The cupula, like the tectorial membrane, is extremely sensitive to the alterations in its ionic environment. The cupula extends to the roof and lateral walls of the ampulla and is firmly attached to crista. The rest of dome of ampulla also contains a loose fibrillar meshwork, but there appears to be space between the cupula and the surface of the crista. The cilia of the sensory cells protrude into this and the longest cilia appear to enter the cupula.

It seems likely that during the angular acceleration the cupula remains fixed and the angle of the junction of semicircular duct and the ampulla, along with the loose matrix within the dome of ampulla, serve to direct endolymph into the subcupular space where the deflection of ciliary bundle occurs, resulting in stimulation or inhibition of the neural output of the sensory cells (Dohlman, 1981).[5] The semicircular canals are not gravity sensitive and cupula does not exert a resting force on the underlying sensory epithelium.

In each macula of utricle and saccule, there is neural epithelium with vestibular sensory cells. A gelatinous material overlies the sensory cells, the ciliary bundles of which appear to project into a honeycomb meshwork in its undersurface. Embedded in the upper surface of the gelatinous layer are the otoconia, which are rich in calcium crystals. These have a characteristic shape with a barrel-shaped body and pointed ends. The term "otoconial membrane" is used to describe the otoconia and the gelatinous membrane. Maculae are gravity-sensitive; respond to linear acceleration and some low frequency acoustic stimulation.

The vestibular sensory epithelium has two types of cells. Type I is a large goblet-shaped cell while type II is cylindrical shaped. From the thickened cuticular plate at the top of the cells protrudes one Kinocillium and 20-100 Stereocilia. The location of Kinocillium gives polarity to the cell. The bending in the direction of kinocillia increases the resting output of the nerve impulses of the afferent neurons while the deflection away decreases the resting discharge.

In BPPV, the well-known pathology of Cupulolithiasis occurs. Histopathological observations of the posterior canal crista in patients of BPPV reveal basophilic deposits embedded into the cupula of the posterior semicircular canal of the undermost ear in the provocation position. Presumably, these deposits are derived from the otoconial blanket located over the utricular macula. This otoconia are thought to be dislodged from the utricular macula as a result of head trauma, acute or chronic inflammatory conditions, ageing, or surgical insult to the labyrinth. The otoconia are dislodged and settle in the most dependent part of the labyrinth, i.e. cupula of the posterior semicircular canal. This adhesion of otoconial particles makes the cupula gravity sensitive. This anomalous stimulation causes the positional vertigo in the offending head position.

As opposed to cupulolithiasis, there is also a hypothesis of canalithiasis, i.e. free-floating particles. According to this theory, dense particles, most likely displaced otoconia, collect in the most dependent portion of the endolymphatic system, i.e. the long arm of posterior semicircular canal. It is proposed that the particles dislodged from utricular maculae travel via the crus commune to reach the long arm of semicircular canal. The posterior semicircular canal being the most dependent, the particles gravitate in this canal. According to Epley (1996),[7] the change in position of head causes the free-floating canaliths to gravitate longitudinally through the canal. This simulates a leaking piston and creates a hydrodynamic drag in the canal in downward direction. The effect of this is potentiated by the canal-cupola cross sectional differential. After several seconds of latency required in overcoming the inertia of the entire fluid loop in addition to cupular resistance, cupular displacement occurs, evoking severe nystagmus and vertigo. When the canaliths reach the limit of their descent, the drag ceases, bringing the nystagmus to an abrupt stop. When the head maneouvre is reversed. The particles gravitate in reverse direction. This produces nystagmus in same axis but reverse direction. On repetitive head maneouvres the particles get dispersed and their capability to induce vertigo and nystagmus is reduced progressively.

The hypothesis of canalithiasis is supported by clinical observations. If the heavy cupula theory were correct, the vertigo would be persistent, mild and in the plane of semicircular canal when cupula is horizontally oriented.

CLINICAL PICTURE

The patients present with the history of severe attacks of vertigo in a particular position of head. Sometimes, they get up from sleep at night with severe spinning of head. When this occurs repeatedly, they find themselves in same position of head in bed. This may also occur when they first lie in bed or roll over to one side or other. Mild nausea may occur. Vomiting is not common but can be seen in initial phases. There is no loss of consciousness. Patients feel weak and insecure after an attack but there is no paralysis of limbs. The attacks decrease in frequency over a course of week or month.

The ear nose throat examination is normal. The neurological examination is negative. The audiological examination and electronystagmography may be normal. CAT scan and/or MRI for brain maybe done in selected cases to allay the anxiety of the patient. The scans are normal. In some cases, cervical spondylitis is seen. There is no correlation between BPPV and cervical spondylitis. The diagnostic test is a positive positional test. The test for positional nystagmus is described as follows.

Examination for Positional Nystagmus

The examination for positional nystagmus is done as shown in Fig. 3.2. To simplify the examination; positional nystagmus is sought in second-degree position, i.e. looking straight ahead. The patient is asked to lie on a couch or a table. He is then told to look straight ahead. Using a head mirror inverted at the top of examiner's head and asking the patient to look at the hole in the mirror helps the patient in following instructions. The examiner should keep his head in front of the patient when looking for nystagmus. The patient should be told that his head will be held in various positions and that it is important that he keeps his eyes open and tells if he feels an attack of vertigo. He is also instructed not to try to change his position when vertigo occurs. He is reassured that the examiner will ensure his security and that in most cases the attack will subside in a minute or two. At first, look for any spontaneous nystagmus. Then the examiner who stands behind the patient holds the patient's head. The patient is then put rapidly in supine position with the head hanging below the edge of the table. If there is no nystagmus in 60 seconds, the patient is taken to the sitting position again. The same procedure is repeated

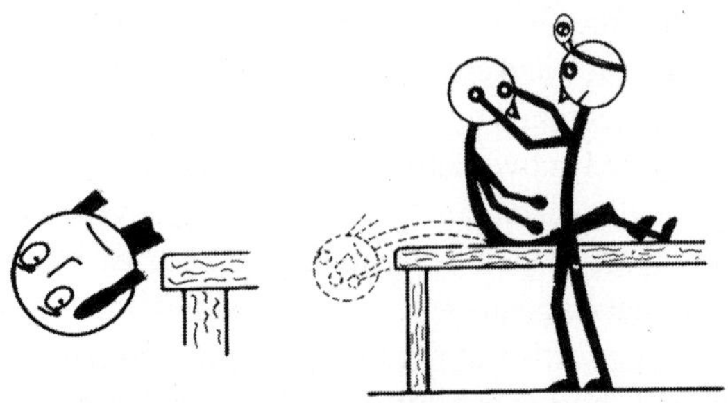

Fig. 3.2: Showing the positional test procedure

with the patient's head in left and then right lateral position with head hanging down. In a positive response, the vertigo and nystagmus appear in 2-20 seconds. Patient's head is retained in the offending position until the vertigo and nystagmus subside. However, if the nystagmus persists beyond 60 seconds, it is recorded as being persistent. On repeating the tests, the vertigo and nystagmus may not appear every time and it may be less intense.

The BPPV has to be differentiated from more serious central type of vertigo. The central lesion is mostly of tumours involving the CP angle, cerebellum, and pontine lesion. Harrison and Ozsahinoglu (1972)[10] found in 1% cases of proven central lesions the presence of a peripheral type of positional nystagmus. Table 3.1 shows the salient differences in a benign peripheral and more serious central positional nystagmus. Thus, it is important that a serious central lesion should be excluded by neurological examination and if needed a CAT scan or an MRI of brain.

Table 3.1: Showing differences between peripheral and central nystagmus

Characteristics	*Peripheral*	*Central*
Latency	2-20 seconds	None
Persistence	Disappears in 60 sec	Persists
Fatigability	Present	Absent
Position	One position only	Multiple
Vertigo	Always present	Sometimes only
Direction of nystagmus	One fixed	Changing
Incidence	85%	15%

Treatment

The treatment of such patients can best be discussed as medical, surgical, physiotherapy and canalith repositioning maneouvres. The canaliths repositioning maneuvers are the most accepted method of treatment.

Medical Treatment

This aspect is dependent on use of vestibular sedatives, i.e. Prochlorperazine or tranquilizers, i.e. Diazepam or vestibular sedatives with vasodilator properties, i.e. Cinnerazine. Non-sedating antivertiginous drugs like betahistine are preferred as they aid in habituation. The results as regards symptom control are good but drugs have to be taken for a long time. The medicines do not tackle the problem of canaliths, but as the disease is self-limiting, patients are able to lead normal life with reassurance and explanation of the aetiology.

Surgical Treatment

The surgical treatment is only rarely required as most cases can be controlled by medical treatment. Two main treatment approaches are the denervation of posterior semicircular canal by singular neurectomy (Gacek, 1985)[8] and posterior canal occlusion (Parnes and McClure, 1990).[15] There are a number of modifications to the original technique (Parnes, 1996).[16] Majority of patients benefit from surgery. The surgery should, however, be limited to a very few patients who cannot be controlled by other means and are so miserable that they request for it. There were concerns expressed that the surgery of posterior canal may lead to increased sensorineural hearing loss. Labyrinthectomy and vestibular nerve section cure the patients of BPPV. The labyrinthectomy is associated with total hearing loss.

Physiotherapy

Head and balance excersises described by Cawthorne and Cooksey or one of their numerous modifications, helps in improving the balance. Habituation occurs in majority of cases. They should be recommended to the patients of BPPV.

Canalith Repositioning Procedure

Epley (1992)[6] developed the canalith repositioning procedure (CRP). The procedure is now widely accepted as a treatment of choice in cases of BPPV.

Rationale

The objective of the CRP is to move the canaliths out of the canal to the utricle, where they will no longer affect the canal dynamics. Head maneouvres rotate the target canal while keeping its orientation coplanar with the gravity, thereby inducing the canaliths to migrate through gravitation away from the ampulla. The procedure described here can be conducted on a simple examination table. It is not ideal but has proved effective in clinical settings.

Simultaneously, the induced nystagmus can be tracked to study the direction and rate of canalith migration. This is best accomplished by direct observation. The eyelids should be lifted up to further expose sclera as it provides for an observation with better global perspective of the torsional movement. The Frenzel's glasses are not of help as visual fixation is not a problem. The recording by electronystagmography or video-oculography can be helpful.

A timing strategy is combined with the positioning sequence to control the rotation rate so that the gravitating canaliths are kept in the portion of the canal, which is vertically oriented at the moment. This keeps them constantly moving towards utricle. The duration of nystagmus is directly related to the movement of the particles, thus each movement duration is determined by the duration of the nystagmus. It is important that each step should achieve the rotation of the canal through approximately 90-degrees or less because the canaliths can gravitate through approximately 90-degree segment only at a time when the canal is held steady.

An oscillating device can be applied to the skull throughout the procedure to minimise the adherence of the canaliths to the canal wall. However, acceptable results can be obtained without this modification.

Procedure

The first step is to identify the offending posterior semi-circular canal. It is the lowermost canal in the offending head position. The latency and duration of the induced nystagmus are noted to assess the duration for which the canal has to be maintained in a given position.

Preparation

The patient is premedicated with 5 mg diazepam or transdermal scopolamine on the night before the test. The ENG electrodes are applied and the patient is put on the examining table in the supine position so that when lying down, the head of the patient should protrude beyond the table.

Maneouvres

The positioning sequence is shown in Fig. 3.3. The appropriate positioning sequence is commenced. If nystagmus is induced from one position to next, the slowing of nystagmus is taken to indicate that the canalith bolus has reached the end of descent. The head is then

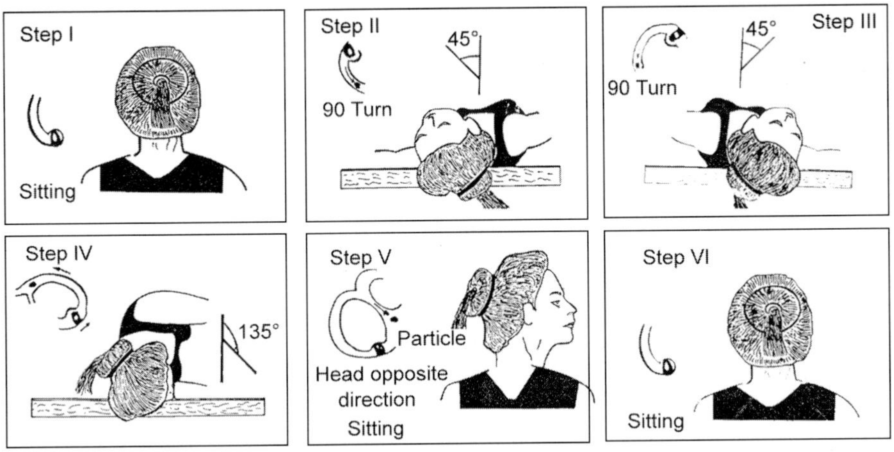

Fig. 3.3: Showing particle repositioning maneouvre

maneouvred to next position. Typical time in each position is 6-13 seconds but can be as much as 30 seconds. If no nystagmus is observed, the duration as calculated from the positional test is used to adjust the timing. The nystagmus may not occur at times because the canaliths are so much dispersed for nystagmus to be elicited. The sequence is repeated until no nystagmus appears or no progress is apparent in last two cycles.

Oscillation

An oscillator with 80 Hz vibrations is held throughout against the hand of the examiner kept on mastoid process of the skull throughout the procedure.

Follow-up

Patients are advised to avoid head back and head forwards procedure for 48 hrs after a treatment session. The CRP is repeated at weekly intervals until the nystagmus completely dissappears. The CRP is also stopped if no further progress occurs on CRP maneouvres.

Anticipated Results

Ninety per cent of patients should have complete relief of symptoms and negative Dix- Hallpike tests. If the CRP is not properly performed, the results are suboptimal.

Precautions

Care should be taken with patients who have cervical spondylosis or any other disease like retinal detachment likely to be aggravated by cervical movements or vibrator. In some cases sudden rapid nystagmus may occur. This could be due to jamming of the canaliths. It can be reversed by moving the head by 180 degrees. The oscillator helps in dislodging the otoliths, which sometimes become jammed.

No serious complications have been encountered in a large number of cases where the CRP has been carried out. Rarely the particles may go in wrong direction and to another canal. If they enter the lateral semicircular canal, suitable repositioning maneouvres can be used.

A careful examination should always be done to exclude any ear disease causing vertigo.

Benign Positional Vertigo of Chidhood

Herraiz *et al* (1999)[11] have reported benign positional vertigo in childhood (BPVC). They have postulated a common pathway for migraine and BPVC based on ischaemia due to vasoconstriction secondary to abnormal accumulation of vasoactive substances (seratonin and prostaglandins).

Summary

BPPV is a common diagnosis in cases of vertigo. The diagnosis is based on positive test for positional vertigo. All other examinations are normal. The investigations can be done to exclude any other disease of ear or central nervous system. The investigations are rarely required.

The treatment of choice is the canaliths (particle) repositioning maneouvres.

The medical treatment and physiotherapy suffice for a number of cases.

The surgical treatment is for a very small number of refractory cases that are unable to lead normal life on medicines, particle repositioning and physiotherapy.

Results of treatment are good and Otolaryngologists should give excellent prognosis to patients of BPPV.

REFERENCES

1. Barany R, Diagnose von krankheitsercheinungen im bereiche des otolithenapparetes. Acta Otolaryngol. (Stockh) 1921; 2:434-37.
2. Barber HO. Positional nystagmus. In New York, Academic press, "The vestibular system", Naunton (Ed) 1975; 303-19.
3. Barber HO. Positional nystagmus—Testing and interpretation. Ann. Otol 1964; 73: 838-50.
4. Dix MR and Hallpike CS. The pathology, symptomatology and diagnosis of certain common disorders of the vestibular system. Ann. Otol 1952, 61: 987-1016.
5. Dohlman CF. Critical review of the concept of cupula function. Acta. Otolaryngologica. Supplementum 1981; 376, 1-6.
6. Epley JM, Benign paroxysmal positional vertigo: New methods of diagnosis and management. In Johnson, JT, Derkay, CS, Mandell-brown, MK, Newman RK (Eds): Instructional Courses Vol. 5, St Louis: Mosby-yearbook, 1992.
7. Epley JM. Particle repositioning for benign paroxysmal positional vertigo. Otolaryngological Clinics of North America 1996; 29:323-31.
8. Gacek RR. Pathophysiology and management of cupulolithiasis. American Journal of Otolaryngology, 1985; 5: 66-74.
9. Grace RR. Pathology of the vestibular system in Scott-Brown's otolaryngology. In Booth JB (ed) Otology 126-55, Butterworth International edition, 1987.
10. Harrison MS and Ozsahinoglu C. Positional vertigo: Etiology and clinical significance. Brain 1972; 95: 369-72.
11. Herraiz C, Calvin FJ, Tapia MC, Lucas PD and Arroyo R. The migraine: Benign paroxysmal vertigo of childhood complex. The international tinnitus journal 1999; 5: 50-52.
12. Morales-Garcia C and Goycoolea M. Benign paroxysmal vertigo in Modern concepts of neuro-otology. Ed Sandra Desa Souza and Claus Claussen : Prajakta arts, India, 1997, 247-66.
13. Morales-Garcia C. Cochleo-vestibular involvement in otosclerosis. Acta. Otolaryngol. (Stockh) 1972; 73:484-92.
14. Nylen CO. A clinical study on positional nystagmus in cases of brain tumor: Acta. Otolaryngology. (Stockh), 1931; Suppl. 15.
15. Parnes LS and McClure JA. Posterior semicircular canal occlusion for intractable benign paroxysmal positional vertigo. Ann. Otol. Rhinol. Laryngol. 1990; 99: 330-34.
16. Parnes LS. Update on posterior canal occlusion for benign paroxysmal positional vertigo. Otolaryngologic Clinics of North America 1996; 333-41.

CHAPTER 4

Surgical Treatment of Vertigo

Nikita S. Malhotra, Santosh K. Kacker,
Milind V. Kirtane

Vertigo can be a disabling symptom and the patient so incapacitated, that surgery is almost demanded. By 'incapacitated' one implies that the symptoms are still present after adequate medical evaluation and treatment. It is understood, therefore, that these surgeries are performed in a small percentage of patients, since in the majority of cases, medical treatment alone will suffice. None of the many surgical procedures available are universally accepted or provide 100% relief. These are the factors to keep in mind when selecting a specific approach. In addition, it should be kept in mind that vertigo is a manifestation of an underlying problem that must be assessed and (if possible) defined; and depending on the cause, different surgical alternatives will be selected.

On a pragmatic basis, we can classify conditions that cause vertigo that may require surgical intervention, according to whether they occur in the middle ear, inner ear or internal acoustic meatus. There is also another group of conditions, such as vertebrobasilar insufficiency and subclavian steal syndrome, in which surgical correction of the vascular obstruction may relieve vertigo.

We will restrict ourselves to surgical procedures designed for treatment of vertigo of labyrinthine origin. The most common peripheral labyrinthopathy for which surgery is advised is Meniere's disease. The other conditions are benign positional paroxysmal vertigo (BPPV), spontaneous perilymph fistula and vascular loops pressing on the VIIIth cranial nerve. Otosclerosis, vestibular neuronitis, posterior fossa tumours and labyrinthitis due to otitis media can also manifest as vertigo.

The surgeries described here are classified according to the anatomical structure being addressed.

SURGERY FOR MENIERE'S DISEASE

A. Operations on the Endolymphatic Sac

1. Endolymphatic sac decompression / Enhancement
2. Endolymphatic-mastoid shunt
3. Endolymphatic-subarachnoid shunt

B. Operations to Create Fistulae or Shunts in the Labyrinth

1. Sacculotomy
   - Fick procedure
   - Cody 'tack' procedure
2. Cochleosacculotomy
3. Utriculostomy
4. Stapedectomy-sacculotomy
5. Others
   - Fistulisation of the lateral semicircular canal
   - Otic periotic shunt

C. Destruction of the Vestibular End Organ

1. Chemical labyrinthectomy
   - Gentamicin
   - Streptomycin
2. Surgical labyrinthectomy
   - Transtympanic labyrinthectomy
   - Transmastoid labyrinthectomy
   - Labyrinthectomy through the middle fossa
3. Ultrasonic irradiation of the labyrinth
4. Cryosurgery

D. Vestibular Nerve Section

- Through the middle fossa
- Retrolabyrinthine
- Retrosigmoid
- Translabyrinthine

E. Miscellaneous Procedures

- Sympathectomy
- Ventilation tube placement

A. OPERATIONS ON THE ENDOLYMPHATIC SAC

1. Endolymphatic Sac Decompression/Enhancement

This procedure is oriented towards relieving endolymphatic hydrops that is presumably responsible for precipitating vertigo in Meniere's disease. The original endolymphatic sac drainage procedure was first described by Portmann in 1926. It is remarkable that Portmann's procedure based on his interpretation of pathogenesis, preceded histological confirmation of endolymphatic hydrops by 12 years and it is still the most commonly performed operation for Meniere's disease although many modifications have evolved. The aim of the operation is to enhance the drainage of the endolymph by relieving congestion and pressure. This involves decompression of the labyrinth at the level of the endolymphatic sac, and thus at a distance of more than 1 cm from the sensory organelles of the labyrinth.

The surgery can be performed under local anaesthesia. A postauricular transmastoid approach is used. A cortical mastoidectomy is performed, the horizontal semicircular canal identified at the base of the antrum and followed posteriorly without blue lining it. The posterior semicircular canal is then located usually about 2 mm farther medially than the lateral border of the horizontal canal. The sigmoid sinus is further identified. If it is anteriorly placed and obstructing access to the Trautmann's triangle, it is burred down until a small blade can be inserted to retract the sinus posteriorly during dissection of the endolymphatic sac. Next, the posterior fossa dural plate between the sigmoid sinus and posterior semicircular canal is removed. The bony posterior semicircular canal is gently blue lined to its lowest point inferiorly. Also, the bone at the posterior surface of the pyramid is thinned adequately till the dura is just visible through the bone. In a well-pneumatised petrous bone, the upper border of the endolymphatic sac is visible under the dura as a whitish area with well-defined upper margins, just behind the inferior half of the posterior semicircular canal. Alternatively, the Donaldsen's line can be used for identification. It is an imaginary line drawn from the horizontal semicircular canal along its longitudinal axis, bisecting the posterior canal and passing up to the sigmoid sinus. The top of the sac is located here in the posterior fossa dura (Fig. 4.1).

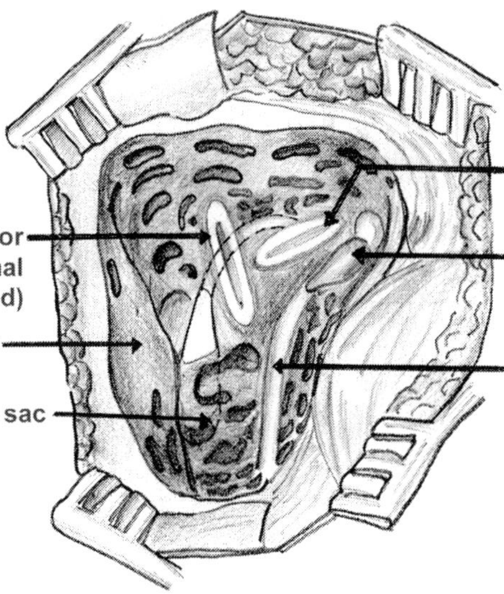

Fig. 4.1: Endolymphatic sac decompression

With the help of smaller diamond burrs, bone behind as well as inferior to the blue line of the posterior semicircular canal is removed and the pale upper border and lateral surface of the endolymphatic sac is traced. The sac is a pear shaped, thickened, white, shiny, double-layered structure. Burring is done gently at the junction of the petrous bone and endolymphatic sac. The sac is then followed laterally and partially separated from the dura. The lateral wall of the sac is then incised and a piece of silicon film cut to a sharp angle is inserted into the lumen. The sac and the film are further covered with a connective tissue graft taken from behind the auricle.

Alternatively, 1-2 silastic T-struts are placed in the sac. The tail of the strut is placed outside the sac between the dura and bone to decompress the dura and continguous lateral sinus permanently. T-struts within the lumen enlarge the lumen and help passive transfer of endolymph.

A silastic apron is placed to cover this region followed by 1 or 2 large pieces of gelfoam dipped in sterile antibiotic solution. The wound is then closed in layers.

A ventilation tube may be placed in the tympanic membrane and middle ear suctioned through this site, which facilitates drainage of operated fluids from the middle ear and mastoid in the immediate postoperative period; and also promotes middle ear and mastoid ventilation via an enlarged aditus.

Complications include bleeding from the lateral sinus, if anteriorly placed. Due to inadvertent incision of dura, there is a likelihood of a CSF fistula. A small such defect can be repaired by plugging with connective tissue. Facial nerve damage may also occur. Patient may suffer from a severe sensorineural hearing loss or dead ear (2-5%), due to infection which may lead to scarring immediately over the sac or spread of infection to the labyrinth. A foreign body granuloma must be suspected if the patient presents with rapidly progressive hearing loss and/or nystagmus 2-5 days postoperatively. Treatment is by re-exploration. The patient may also have recurrence of symptoms such as vertigo due to postauricular depression of the wound and bone and scar tissue growing into the extrasaccular region causing obstruction.

Overall improvement rate of 65-70 per cent has been noted after surgery in the various studies undertaken. However, these procedures have the advantage of being conservative, low-risk and effective procedures, which if necessary, can also be revised and additionally allow the performance of any other surgical alternative.

2. Endolymphatico-Mastoid Shunt

This is achieved by exposing the sac as mentioned above. A silastic strip, drain or absorbable gelatin film is placed in the lumen of the sac and the lateral wall of the sac is folded back. The pitfall of this procedure is invasion of the sac by fibrosis or granulation tissue from the mastoid.

3. Endolymphatico-Subarachnoid Shunt

This is done by placing a small incision on the medial surface of the sac in order to open up the subarachnoid space. Into this opening, a flanged teflon tube preferably with a unidirectional valve is inserted. The flange stays in the lumen of the sac and prevents displacement of the shunt. Whenever the endolymph pressure rises, the shunt permits its drainage into the subarachnoid space.

No significant difference between the above procedures was noted in the control of vertigo or the stabilisation of hearing. Successful resolution of vertigo occurred in less than 60 per cent of cases.

B. OPERATIONS TO CREATE FISTULAE OR SHUNTS IN THE LABYRINTH

1. Sacculotomy

This procedure is meant to decompress the endolymphatic system by a puncture of the dilated saccule through the footplate of the stapes, which relieves perilymph pressure and, in turn, endolymph pressure in the saccule. Two techniques have been described, both using a permeatal approach and raising a tympanomeatal flap.

The Fick operation involves piercing the dilated saccule through the footplate with the help of a sharp pick. Gelatin sponge or connective tissue is then used to cover the fenestra in the oval window. Reported relief of vertigo with this procedure is 70-90 per cent.

The Cody 'tack' procedure attempts to create a more permanent fistula in the saccule by permanently placing a tack through the fenestra in the footplate. Improvement has been noted in 65-70% of patients.

These procedures often lead to severe, irreversible sensorineural hearing loss and hence have not found widespread acceptance. They are mentioned here for the sake of completeness and an overall concept.

2. Cochleosacculotomy

This procedure was developed by Schucknecht in 1982. The purpose is to create an endocochlear fistula through which excess endolymph can drain into the perilymph space. This procedure is performed under local anaesthesia. A tympanomeatal flap is elevated to gain adequate exposure of the oval and round windows. The superior lip of the round window niche is drilled away with a small cutting burr, allowing visualisation of the round window membrane. A 3 mm right-angled pick is introduced through the round window membrane in the direction of the oval window and pushed to its full depth, thus piercing the spiral lamina and establishing a permanent connection with the vestibule, creating an endolymphatic-perilymphatic shunt. This simple procedure gives relief from vertigo in about 70-75% of patients but carries an inherent risk of hearing loss, especially for high frequencies. It should be reserved for cases with poor hearing where labyrinthectomy may not be desirable, especially in elderly or disabled patients.

3. Utriculostomy

This is a new alternative still in an experimental stage. It involves making a permanent fistula in the membranous labyrinth (utricle) and establishing a connection between the endolymphatic and perilymphatic space. This has been achieved experimentally (in sheep) through the oval window with microcauterisation using radio frequency. Advantages of this procedure are permanent communication (in contrast to puncture), avoidance of altering the saccule (with inherent hearing loss) and simplicity of surgical approach (exploratory tympanotomy – oval window approach). Clinical documentation in humans is still awaited.

4. Stapedectomy-Sacculotomy

This is reserved for patients in whom otosclerosis and Meniere's disease coexist. In these cases, a stapedectomy is followed by replacement using a wire and connective tissue prosthesis, 4.5 mm long, which has a small peg. In order to encourage saccular decompression, the sharpened tip of the wire protrudes 0.75 to 1 mm below the level of the oval window graft (Fig. 4.2).

C. DESTRUCTION OF THE VESTIBULAR END ORGAN

1. Chemical Labyrinthectomy

Selective destruction of the vestibular labyrinth can be achieved pharmacologically by using vestibulotoxic drugs of the Aminoglycoside group, namely Streptomycin and Gentamicin. Although known to be vestibulotoxic, they are potentially ototoxic. As they can potentially affect the central nervous system pathways, close monitoring is necessary during their administration. These drugs have been used topically in the middle ear or applied to the inner ear via a labyrinthotomy, and systemically to control the symptoms of Meniere's disease.

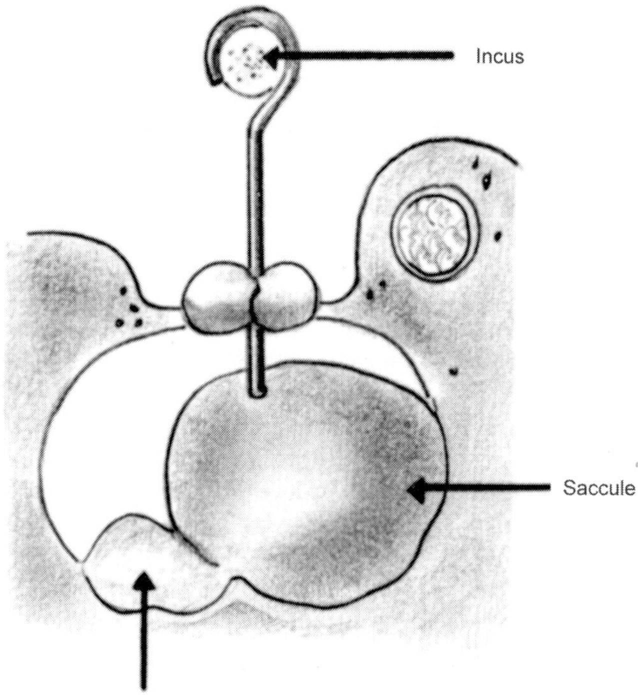

Fig. 4.2: Stapedectomy-sacculotomy

Fowler described chemical labyrinthectomy using Streptomycin in 1948. It is useful to obtain a baseline audiogram and caloric test results prior to initiating treatment. Intramuscular injections of Streptomycin are given in a dose of 1 g, every 8 to 12 hours. Daily audiograms and caloric tests are done. Treatment is continued until caloric response is abolished or there is evidence of ototoxicity such as appearance of tinnitus. The technique of Streptomycin perfusion through the horizontal semicircular canal as described by Shea has the disadvantage of a high incidence of sensorineural hearing loss and hence has not gained popularity.

Intratympanic use of Streptomycin or Gentamicin has been described as an alternate method to achieve selective vestibular ablation. Various techniques and dose schedules to deliver Gentamicin have been described, such as instillation of Gentamicin into the middle ear cavity using polyethylene tubing placed either transmeatally or after an endaural incision; or instillation using a syringe and cannula under an operating microscope. Nedzelski popularised the technique of inserting a tympanostomy tube through the tympanic membrane under local anaesthesia, in the postero-inferior quadrant to a position approximately over the round window area. The tympanostomy tube is connected to plastic tubing through the external ear and sutured preauricularly. A solution containing 26.7 mg/ml of Gentamicin is instilled slowly into the middle ear at a rate of about 1 ml into the middle ear over 10 minutes, with the patient supine and head turned away 45 degrees from the affected ear. The patient remains in this position for 30 minutes to allow pooling of the solution over the round window. Treatment is arrested after 3 injections daily for 4 days or at the onset of vestibular symptoms. Treatment is terminated prematurely if nystagmus is observed, if the patient complains of unsteadiness associated with a deterioration of tandem gait or if a significant decrease in hearing occurs. Follow-up procedures include keeping track of vertigo spells, caloric testing and speech discrimination.

Indications for treatment are active, unilateral Meniere's disease with frequent, disabling attacks of vertigo, which have not responded to conservative medical treatment. Contraindications include a pre-existing tympanic membrane perforation, active inflammation of middle ear, aminoglycoside allergy, impaired renal function, high risk of poor post-procedural central nervous system compensation and Meniere's disease in an only hearing ear. Advantages of this procedure are avoidance of hospitalisation and of severe vertigo, while disadvantages are prolonged treatment with repeated visits and the possibility of recurrence of symptoms, in which case re-treatment may be necessary.

2. Surgical Labyrinthectomy

These procedures are employed to control vertigo in profoundly or totally deafened ears with residual, damaged vestibular function. When these procedures are considered in patients with unilateral non-useful hearing, it is to be kept in mind that Meniere's disease is bilateral in a significant number of cases and that symptoms do not manifest simultaneously in both ears. Therefore, a labyrinthectomy in a patient with unilateral Meniere's disease can be a potential nightmare if the second ear becomes symptomatic and the symptoms incapacitating. The degree and type of destruction is also considered if a cochlear implant is a potential procedure. Relief of vertigo after surgical labyrinthectomy is very good (93-95%).

a. Transtympanic Labyrinthectomy

This procedure is indicated in elderly patients or in patients whom general anaesthesia is hazardous. Advantages of this procedure are that it may be performed under local anaesthesia and requires a short operating time. The ear is opened through an endaural transcanal approach as in stapedectomy. The tympanomeatal flap is raised allowing good exposure of the promontory, oval and round windows. The stapes is then removed following which the bony bridge between the lower part of the oval and round windows is drilled away establishing a broad connection between both windows. Further, the saccular and utricular maculae are removed from the vestibule through the oval window. A 3 mm right-angled hook is then introduced into the vestibule and with a blind sweep, the neuroepithelium is removed from the ampullary cavity of the lateral, superior and posterior canals. The vestibule is aspirated and can be filled with Streptomycin-soaked gelfoam to destroy any residual vestibular function. The labyrinthine defect is closed with fascia or perichondrium and the tympanomeatal flap is returned to position.

b. Transmastoid Labyrinthectomy

This procedure offers the advantage of a more complete removal of vestibular function. A simple mastoidectomy is done and the bony labyrinth exposed. Each of the 3 semicircular canals is individually drilled and the membranous canals are avulsed using a hook. By following the canals to their ampullary ends, the vestibule is widely opened and the neuroepithelium removed from within under direct visualisation.

Vertigo may recur following a technically flawless labyrinthectomy, usually with a latency of months or years resulting from some residual function of vestibular organelles left in the exenterated labyrinth. This may perhaps also occur from some irritation of Scarpa's ganglion. A neurectomy is indicated in these cases.

3. Ultrasonic Irradiation of the Labyrinth

Application of ultrasonic irradiation to the labyrinth has been advocated as a surgical method to ablate vestibular function by destroying the cristae of the semicircular canals while preserving the organ of corti and thus the hearing (selective labyrinthectomy). Ultrasonic energy is applied to the inner ear by placing the source on the thinned otic capsule of the horizontal semicircular canal via a simple mastoidectomy approach, or on the round window via a tympanotomy incision. As the ultrasonic irradiation is absorbed, heat is given off that dissipates quickly through the fluids of the inner ear causing selective injury to the membranous labyrinth. This is associated with a measurable irritative nystagmus for the first half hour, then a period without nystagmus followed by a paralytic nystagmus. Therapy is concluded when no further irritative nystagmus is seen, indicating total ablation.

The initial effects were encouraging, but long-term results have been disappointing with many patients suffering continuous or recurrent vertigo. Vertigo is diminished in approximately 75% of lateral canal procedures and in only 25% of round window procedures.

4. Cryosurgery

This modality is a similar attempt to destroy selectively the vestibular end organ while preserving hearing. It involves transmastoid application of a cryoprobe cooled to –160 °C to the lateral semicircular canal for 3 cycles of 2 minutes each. Hearing is reportedly unaffected by this therapy. Vertigo is controlled in 71-73% of the patients but serious complications of delayed facial paralysis, which occur in 5-8% of these procedures makes it less desirable. As with ultrasonic therapy, a high rate of recurrent vertigo has caused many to abandon this modality.

Another alternative is application of a probe on the promontory, which in turn causes necrosis of the Reissner's membrane in the basal turn of the cochlea. The fistula thus created allows drainage of excess endolymph into the perilymph space.

D. VESTIBULAR NERVE SECTION

Selective sectioning of the vestibular nerve can give excellent relief from vertigo (rates of cure as high as 90%). The nerve can be approached by the middle cranial fossa, the retrolabyrinthine or the retrosigmoid/suboccipital routes. The goals of all 3 techniques are to denervate the vestibular end organ while preserving hearing. The disadvantages of selective vestibular nerve section are incomplete section resulting in sparing of some vestibular fibres. Secondly, the hearing loss may progress as the cochlear pathology remains unaltered, and the feeling of tinnitus and aural fullness may persist. Also, the unacceptably high rates of facial nerve dysfunction and potential risk of neurosurgical complications prevent widespread acceptance of these procedures.

The most common problem treated by neurectomy is Meniere's disease. Other causes of peripheral vestibular dysfunction such as trauma, post-operative damage, uncompensated vestibular neuritis and so forth are also indications for neurectomy. A reproducible and significant decrease in vestibular response on electronystagmographic testing is a valuable pre-operative diagnostic tool for recommendation of a vestibular neurectomy in these other non-Meniere's cases.

1. Transtemporal Vestibular Neurectomy (Sectioning through the middle fossa)

This procedure is done under general anaesthesia. A vertical, slightly curvilinear incision, 8-10 cm long is made, starting anterior to the tragus and over the root of the zygoma towards the vertex. The temporalis fascia is incised followed by a vertical incision of the temporalis muscle. Following outline of an inferiorly based muscle flap at the base (to cover the craniotomy subsequently), a free temporalis muscle graft is harvested for closure of internal auditory canal later on. Periostium from the petrous squama is stripped, a 2.5 × 3.5 cm craniotomy is outlined anteriorly over the root of the zygomatic arch and the bone flap elevated. Dura from the floor of the middle fossa is gently elevated and posterior dissection is carried out till the posterior margin of the superior petrosal sinus. Next, the dura is elevated anteriorly to near the foramen spinosum and medially above the greater and lesser petrosal nerves.

After the floor of the middle fossa is exposed, the blue line of the superior semicircular canal is identified. An area of meatal plane medial to the superior canal is burred open and the dura of the internal auditory canal identified. The course of the internal auditory meatus is then determined by appropriate bone removal. Next, Bill's bar is identified, anterior to which the facial nerve enters the fallopian canal in the superior part of the fundus of the internal auditory meatus. Posterior to the facial nerve is the superior vestibular nerve. Dura over the superior vestibular nerve is incised and the nerve mobilised and progressively sectioned medial to Scarpa's ganglion. The internal auditory canal defect is covered with the temporalis muscle graft taken earlier. The temporal bone flap is replaced and the antero-inferiorly based temporalis muscle flap is swung into the lower part of the craniotomy. The wound is closed in layers.

Complications include CSF leak, extracranial or intracranial haematoma, transient facial palsy and secondary infection. Success rate of 90-95% is reported in controlling vertigo. Hearing is preserved in about 75% cases.

2. Retrolabyrinthine Vestibular Neurectomy

This is the most widely used approach. It entails a complete mastoidectomy with identification of lateral and posterior semicircular canals. Following decompression of the sigmoid sinus and removal of posterior fossa dura from the bone, the cerebello-pontine angle is entered by creating a flap of dura that is draped over the posterior semicircular canal. The mobile sigmoid sinus and cerebellum are retracted, the VIIth and VIIIth nerve complex identified and the superior half of the VIIIth nerve complex is sectioned. Rate of success in controlling vertigo is 90-95% with decreased risk of complications.

This procedure is indicated for patients with disabling vertigo and normal or aidable hearing. It can also be done for failed endolymphatic sac procedures.

3. Retrosigmoid Vestibular Neurectomy

This procedure is recently introduced in an attempt to identify the vestibular nerves in a more lateral position after their division from the cochlear nerve, thus accomplishing a more complete section. In this approach, the cerebello-pontine angle is entered posterior to the sigmoid sinus through a craniotomy opening. The posterior lip of the internal auditory canal (IAC) is drilled away until the singular canal is identified (inferior aspect). The superior vestibular nerve is sectioned as well as the posterior ampullary nerve. The remaining inferior vestibular nerve fibres are not transected, as they are intimately associated with the cochlear nerve.

4. Translabyrinthine Cochleo-vestibular Neurectomy

In this procedure, a cortical mastoidectomy is performed. Next, the horizontal, posterior and superior semicircular canals are opened and their course identified. The fundus of the IAC is projected between the opened superior and posterior ampullae. The endolymphatic duct is visualised in the bone on the posterior wall of the pyramid. The facial nerve must be skeletonised to approach and expose the fundus of the IAC. Also, the same purpose is served by widely excavating the sinodural angle superiorly and posteriorly. Access to the posterior semicircular canal ampulla is established by removal of bone between the inferior part of mastoid portion of the facial nerve and the anterior border of the sigmoid sinus. Bone removal medial to this ampulla exposes the singular nerve, which enters the IAC fundus in a thin bony canal. Next, the dura on the posterior wall of the IAC is broadly separated from the bone up to the roof and down to the floor of the canal. The dura is incised and partially resected to expose the vestibular nerve. The peripheral portion of the superior vestibular nerve and the inferior vestibular nerve branches are mobilised and the vestibulofacial anastomosis divided. The vestibular nerve is sectioned medial to the Scarpa's ganglion. The facial nerve courses above the transverse crest and the cochlear nerve below it. The cochlear nerve is divided near the fundus of the IAC, thus disrupting the cochlear pathways. The IAC is closed with a small, postauricular free muscle graft. The wound is closed in layers.

Complications include a CSF leak and facial nerve palsy.

E. MISCELLANEOUS PROCEDURES

1. Sympathectomy

The aim of this procedure is to interrupt the distribution of the sympathetic nervous system to the head, thus enhancing the blood supply to the labyrinth. The main indication is for patients with bilateral disease in which the better ear is believed to be the one, which is active in causing symptoms. This procedure can be done bilaterally leading to freedom of vertigo or at least a decrease in frequency and intensity of recurrent episodes. The autonomic nervous system is believed by some to play a role in the pathogenesis of Meniere's disease, probably due to excessive endolymphatic secretion. A Stellate ganglion block may precede this procedure.

The sympathectomy technique includes exposure of the cervical chain and uncovering of that portion from the third thoracic ganglion to just above the Stellate ganglion. However, this operation has the disadvantage of causing bilateral Horner's syndrome, and regeneration of sympathetic trunk may occur.

2. Ventilation Tube Placement

Placement of a ventilation tube in the tympanic membrane was first advocated by Tumarkin, based on the theory that pressure variation in the middle ear plays a triggering role in episodes of vertigo. Control of vertigo in approximately 85-90% of patients has been reported, although more controlled studies are being carried out to ascertain and assess the efficacy of this treatment.

SURGERY FOR BENIGN PAROXYSMAL POSITIONAL VERTIGO (BPPV)

BPPV is one of the common causes of episodic vertigo seen in neuro-otologic practice. It is thought to be caused by high specific gravity deposits in the cupula (cupulolithiasis), or membranous posterior semicircular canal (canalolithiasis) as a result of trauma, ageing, viral infection or surgical insult to the middle ear. The vast majority of patients (90%) undergo spontaneous resolution or cure by adaptation exercises or particle repositioning maneouvres such as Epley's and Semont's techniques which are designed to dislodge the otoconial debris. The very small number of patients with disabling chronic paroxysmal positional vertigo (more than 1 year duration) can be effectively relieved (in 95% of cases) by surgery. Since the pathology involves the ampulla of the posterior semicircular canal, surgery is aimed at selective denervation (singular neurectomy), or plugging the canal to isolate it.

1. Singular Neurectomy

The singular nerve, which is a branch of the inferior vestibular nerve, supplies the ampulla of the posterior semicircular canal. The procedure involves a transcanal approach under local anaesthesia and raising a tympanomeatal flap. Bony overhang of the round window niche is fully removed to expose the round window membrane. The singular canal is then approached by drilling inferior to the attachment of the round window membrane within the floor of the niche. The posterior ampullary (singular) nerve is identified at a depth of 1.5-2 mm and removed using a small hook (Fig. 4.3).

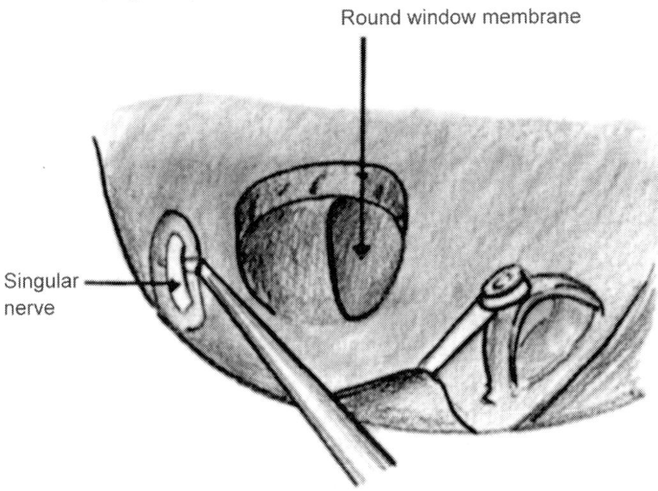

Fig. 4.3: Singular neurectomy

Section of the singular nerve has been reported to give very satisfactory results in treating intractable BPPV. Major disadvantages are significant risk of sensorineural hearing loss (in 3% of patients) and the technically difficult approach with inability to identify the nerve.

2. Plugging of the Posterior Semicircular Canal

The concept of posterior semicircular canal occlusion showed that plugging a semicircular canal would block its function without interfering with other vestibular receptors. The access is through a transmastoid approach, followed by blue-lining of the posterior semicircular canal. The canal is then opened and plugged with bone chips or connective tissue. An alternate procedure is creating a fibrous band in the inner ear by applying the laser over the blue-lined semicircular canal. This procedure thus ablates posterior semicircular canal function without affecting the function of the remaining labyrinth. Also, it does not cause any permanent hearing loss and is safe and effective in the treatment of BPPV. Disadvantages are that it involves opening the labyrinth, which carries with it the inevitable sequelae of surgical labyrinthitis. Also, in one series, most patients reported some postoperative transient unsteadiness, which lasted up to 4 weeks and a transient mild conductive hearing loss secondary to a middle ear collection, which usually resolved in 4 weeks.

CLOSURE OF PERILYMPH FISTULAE

Perilymph or labyrinthine fistula is a communication between the perilymph space of the inner ear and the middle ear or mastoid. It can be congenital, or acquired due to direct trauma causing subluxation or fracture of the footplate of the stapes, cholesteatoma causing bone erosion, or may be spontaneous as in patients with anatomical variations such as wide cochlear aqueduct. Manifestations include sensorineural hearing loss, severe tinnitus, aural fullness and dysequilibrium which are similar to other conditions like BPPV. The most common sites of leak are usually in the inferior aspect of the round window or around the annular ligament of the oval window. Preoperative ENG evaluation may be helpful, but exploratory tympanotomy is the only way to ascertain the diagnosis. In an acute presentation, conservative treatment with bedrest, head end elevation, laxatives, etc. may be tried.

Early repair of perilymph fistula provides potential benefits of resolution of vestibular symptoms and preservation of existing auditory function. Surgery can be performed under general or local anaesthesia. The transcanal approach is used in a wide, patent external auditory meatus, whereas the postauricular approach is used in a narrow canal or one distorted by a fracture. The postauricular approach allows better view of the anterior tympanic sulcus and harvesting of fascia or cortical bone for possible later use in grafting the drum or reconstructing the ossicular chain. The tympanomeatal flap is elevated and middle ear entered. The ossicular chain is inspected and its integrity gently tested. Excessive mobility suggests a dislocation. The incudo-stapedial joint is closely inspected as it may be well aligned although disrupted. If the incus is massively dislocated, it is removed. If the malleus and stapes are intact, reconstruction is achieved by sculpting the dislocated incus and interposing it between the malleus and stapes. Alternatively, a partial ossicular replacement prosthesis (PORP) may be used when the malleus and stapes are at an unfavourable angle.When the malleus and incus are intact but the stape is fractured or dislocated, a stapedectomy is performed, but only for healed injuries of more than 6 weeks. When the incus and stapes are fractured or dislocated, a total ossicular replacement prosthesis (TORP) is placed over the intact footplate. If the oval window is open, a tissue graft is interposed between the labyrinth and the medial end of the prosthesis.

Both the oval and round windows are inspected for any obvious perilymph leakage. If the leak is seen, the mucosa around the leak is made raw, and the windows then grafted with gelfoam, fat or similar autografting material. If no leak is visualised, provocation by Valsalva's maneouvre, Trendelenberg's positioning or internal jugular vein compression may be tried. In case no leak is found with a presumptive diagnosis of fistula, the round and oval windows are often grafted, as intermittent fistulae have been postulated to occur.

If a fistula of the oval window is found in a post-stapedectomy patient, the prosthesis may be removed but the graft should be left in place. The area around the fistula and grafted material is freshened and denuded. A new tissue graft is then placed and a new prosthesis placed if possible. Postoperative complications include partial or complete sensorineural hearing loss, meningitis and facial paralysis.

Postoperative care is directed at maintaining the integrity of the graft. Patients are instructed to avoid lifting weights, strain and activities that place the head in a dependent position (thus preventing increase in intracranial pressure). A stool softener and antibiotics are given for the first 10 postoperative days.

In perilymph fistula, vestibular disturbances respond better to surgical repair (94%) than auditory symptoms. Symptomatically, 89-90% incidence of recovery after surgery has been reported in patients with true vertigo, and 84% in patients with true dysequilibrium.

SURGERY FOR DECOMPRESSION OF THE COCHLEO-VESTIBULAR NERVE

Compression of trigeminal, facial and cochleovestibular nerves by a vascular loop has now been accepted as a cause of unpleasant signs and symptoms such as tic douloureux, hemifacial spasm, vertigo and tinnitus. Recent studies have demonstrated that symptoms may result from constant pulsation of the arterial loop over a fibrosed cochleovestibular bundle, causing an ectopic focus of activity in the nerve. The term *cochleovestibular nerve compression syndrome* (CNCS) has been suggested to describe this situation. Because CNCS may present either as intractable positional vertigo or may mimic vestibular Ménière's disease, appropriate preoperative diagnosis is imperative for choosing the procedure and predicting postoperative success.

The surgical approach to microvascular decompression of the VIIIth nerve is similar to that of a cerebellopontine angle lesion. The retromastoid approach and the classic suboccipital approach are described, the former having less morbidity and allowing hearing preservation. Surgery involves separating the offending vascular loop from the nerve and interposing either connective tissue or a small piece of teflon sponge, secured in place by tissue glue. Studies reveal that 73% of patients had total relief of symptoms after decompression.

OTHER PROCEDURES

Surgery for reflexogenic vertigo, such as tensor tympani tendon section for vertigo with eructation and hiccupping; and sinus surgery for sinugenic vertigo syndrome are not clearly established and their existence is questionable. In addition, carotid endarterectomy or section of the dorsal spinal rootlets may be indicated for conditions not directly related to the VIIIth nerve or the inner ear, but thought to be responsible for the vertiginous symptoms.

FURTHER READINGS

1. A new decade of surgery for vertigo. Am J Otol 1981 Apr; 29(4):391-401 : Hughes GB.
2. Ablation therapy in the management of Meniere's disease. Acta Otolaryngol (Stockh) 132:1, 1957 : Schucknecht HF.
3. Assessment of surgical procedures for Meniere's disease. Laryngoscope 1979 May; 89(5 Pt 1):737-47 : Snow JB Jr; Kimmelman CP.
4. Intratympanic gentamicin for control of vertigo in Meniere's disease : vestibular signs that specify completion of therapy. Am J Otol, 20(2): 209-19 1999 Mar : Minor LB.
5. Is there a consensus in perilymph fistula management ? Otolaryngol Head Neck Surg. 102:11, 1990 : Hughes GB, sismanis A, House JW.
6. Long-term efficacy of endolymphatic sac surgery for vertigo in Meniere's disease. Otolaryngol Head Neck Surg 1993 Jul; 109(1):83-7 : Telischi FF, Luxford WM.
7. Long-term results of posterior semicircular canal occlusion for intractable benign paroxysmal positional vertigo. Clin Otolaryngol, 24(4):316-23 1999 Aug : Walsh RM, Bath AP, Cullen JR, Rutka JA.

8. Overall view and rationale for surgical alternatives for incapacitating peripheral vertigo. Otolaryngol Clin North Am 1994 Apr; 27(2):283-300 : GoycooleaMV, Ruah CB, Lavinsky L, Morales Garcia C.
9. Posterior fossa vestibular nerve section for the management of peripheral vertigo. Eur Arch Otorhinolaryngol, 256(5):230-2 1999 : Goksu N, Bayazit Y, BederL.
10. Retrolabyrinthine vestibular nerve section : efficacy in disorders other than Meniere's disease, Laryngoscope 101:523-528, 1991 : Kemink JL, Telian SA, el-Kashlan H, Langman AW.
11. Surgery for non-Meniere's vertigo. Acta Otolaryngol Suppl 1994; 513:37-9 : Benecke JE.
12. Surgery for vertigo on the nonservicable hearing ear : transmastoid labyrinthectomy or translabyrinthine vestibular nerve section. Laryngoscope 1993 Dec; 103(12):1321-5: Langman AWLindeman RC.
13. Surgery for vertigo : update 1985. Am J Otol 1985 Sep; 6(5):423-7 : Hughes GB, Hahn JF.
14. Surgery for vertigo (you don't have to live with it). J Otolaryngol 1981 Oct; 343-58 : Silverstein H.
15. Surgical treatment of vertigo. Acta Otolaryngol Suppl 1995; 519:21-5 : PulecJL.
16. Surgical treatment of vertigo. Acta Otolaryngol suppl 1988; 455:86-9 : Bagger-Sjoback D.
17. Surgical treatment of vertigo. J Otolaryngol 1980 Apr; 9(2):121-6 : Nedzelski JM, Barber HO.
18. Surgical treatment of vertigo with retrolabyrinthine vestibular neurectomy, Laryngoscope 98:835-39, 1988 : Monsel EM, Wiet RJ, Young NM, Kazan RP.
19. Translabyrinthine approach, Otolaryngol Clin N Am 25 : 311-30, 1992 : Brackmann DE, Green JD.
20. Transection of posterior ampullary nerve for the relief of BPPV, Ann Otol Rhinol Laryngol p3: 596-605, 1975: Gacek R.
21. What I think of sac surgery in 1989. Am J Otol 1989 May;10(3):230-3 : Glasscock ME 3d, Jackson CG, Poe Ds, Johnson GD.

CHAPTER

5

Microdebriders in Endoscopic Sinus Surgery

Milind V. Kirtane, Hetal Patel, Sujata Muranjan

Functional endoscopic sinus surgery (FESS) has been a major advance in the field of rhinology. Traditional endonasal surgery always left the surgeon desiring more illumination and better visualisation inside the nose. The nasal endoscopes have overcome these two major shortcomings in that the surgeon can have bright illumination inside the nose, and with the various angles of vision, i.e. 0, 30, 45, 70, 90, 120 degrees, can see clearly all the structures in the nose and paranasal sinuses. Special instruments with different angulations and sizes were needed to access all the nooks and corners of the nasal cavity. Thus, a variety of forceps to suit different situations during surgery were devised and the range of instruments increased rapidly. The concept of "functional" surgery became more and more dominant. This meant that the surgeon needed to remove only the pathological tissue, with minimum damage to the surrounding mucosa, the so-called "mucosa sparing technique". This was difficult to achieve with traditional forceps, as it involved grabbing and pulling the tissue, which invariably meant tearing off of adjacent mucosa. This produced larger raw areas with accompanying problems in healing. The introduction of microdebriders (soft tissue shavers) made it possible for the surgeon to achieve this dream of mucosa sparing surgery. The microdebrider allows the surgeon to be very precise in removing tissue, cutting it cleanly, with minimum bleeding and under clear vision, since the built-in suction channel keeps the field clear of blood and debris. Soon the surgeons were doing more and more dissection with these mirodebriders and now almost the entire procedure of FESS can be done with this device.

The concept of using soft tissue shavers is not new. It has been employed in neurosurgery to debulk tumours such as acoustic neuromas and in arthroscopic procedures to excise cartilage. But it is only since the last six years that these shavers came to be used in FESS. Thus, it is important for the endoscopic sinus surgeon to understand the mechanism of these powered instruments and the areas where they can be usefully and optimally employed, at the same time being aware of the complications produced by them.

EQUIPMENT

The microdebrider consists of a console, a handpiece, a suction channel and the shaver tips.

The *console* (Figs. 5.1 and 5.2) has controls for adjusting the speed and direction of rotation of the motor and is operated with the help of a *footswitch*. The motor can be used in the unidirectional or in the oscillatory mode. Most surgeons prefer the oscillatory mode since it is more effective in cutting soft tissue.

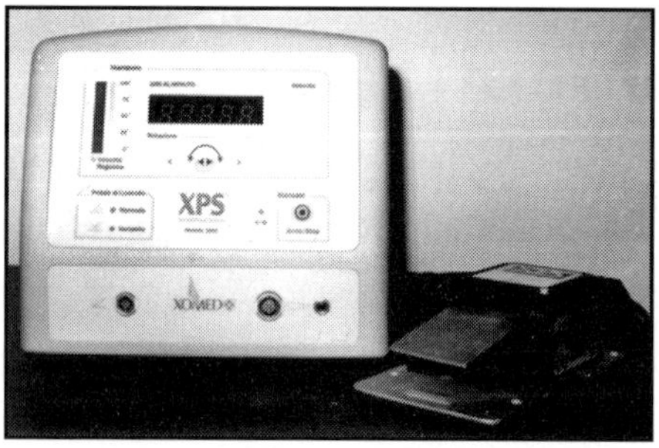

Fig 5.1: Console with footswitch

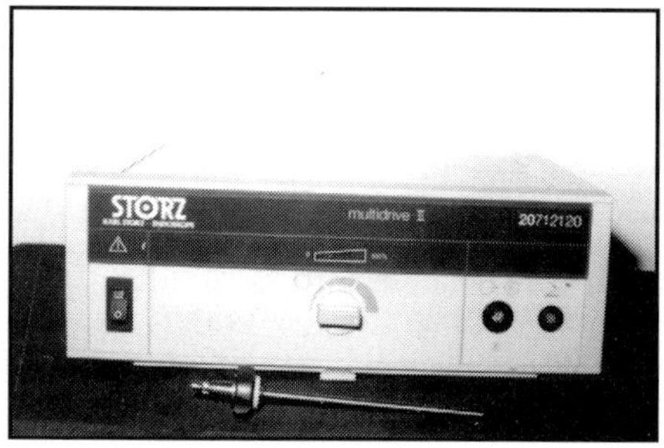

Fig 5.2: Console

The *handpiece* (Fig. 5.3) houses the motor and the suction channel. The shaver blades can be firmly inserted in the distal end of the handpiece.

The *shaver tips* (Fig. 5.3) comprise of an outer cannula and inner blades and are available in various configurations and sizes ranging from 2.5 mm to 5.5 mm diameter. The outer cannula is generally 8 cm in length having a blunt tip and a side eye through which the tissue is sucked in. The rotating inner blade, which is also hollow, has a corresponding side window with cutting edges, which may be straight or serrated. The serrated edges cut larger pieces of tissue while the straight ones are less aggressive and are used in areas where soft tissue needs to be removed off the bone, e.g. over the lamina papyracea. Between the outer cannula and the inner rotating blade, there is a gap of 0.05 mm, which is essential for obtaining a clean cut. The depth of tissue removal is decided by the amount of pressure applied during dissection. The microdebriders with their powerful, in-built suction mechanism have a unique action of simultaneous clean cutting and suctioning of tissues. While the blade cuts only that tissue which has been sucked inside, the blood, bone and tissue debris simultaneously gets sucked away keeping the operating field clean. This permits better visualisation by the surgeon during dissection. Thus, tugging, tearing and avulsion of tissue, which occurs with traditional surgery using forceps is avoided. The efficacy of the entire system depends on the suction, which must be maintained throughout the procedure to prevent clogging. The oscillatory motion of the rotating blade is more effective in cutting tissue than the unidirectional mode. The probable

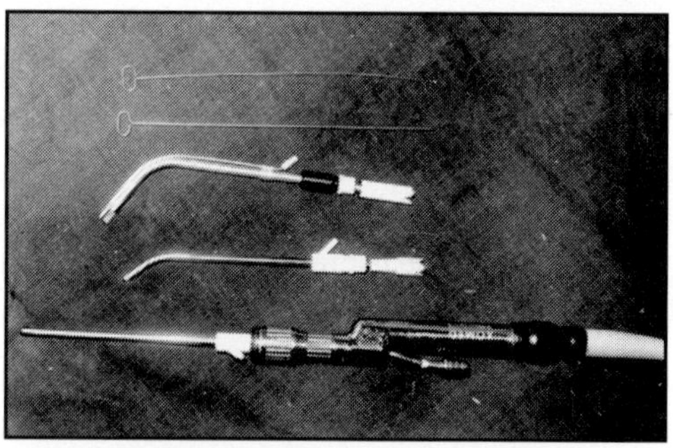

Fig 5.3: Shaver tips with handpiece

reason for this could be that during the unidirectional rotating movement, the tissue tends to get pushed to one side wherein after sometime, the blade merely keeps on touching the tissue but not actually grabbing or cutting it. Whereas with the oscillatory mode, the tissue gets pushed to one side and cut, then immediately pushed the other way as the blade rotates in the reverse direction, thus sucking in more tissue which then gets cut. The speed with which the shaver blades rotate can be controlled from the console wherein the surgeon can adjust the speed to the optimum in a given situation. Most surgeons, however, prefer to operate the microderider at its fastest speed, which in the oscillatory mode is often fixed at 3000 revolution per minute. The blades are also available with the angled tips and can be used in areas such as the frontal recess and within the maxillary sinus. Malleable tips are also available which enable the surgeon to bend them to an angle suitable in a particular situation.

INDICATIONS

In extensive nasal polyposis, where the nostril is completely occluded with polyps, the surgeon encounters difficulty in locating anatomical landmarks at the beginning of surgery. The microdebrider can be used to debulk the polyps with minimum bleeding and minimum trauma to surrounding tissue till the anatomical landmarks such as the middle turbinate and its attachment, the uncinate process and the bulla ethmoidalis become evident. Surgery can then continue with the microdebrider or with traditional instruments as necessary. Other surgical steps can also be performed with the help of the microdebrider. While doing an uncinectomy, one cannot use the shaver right away on the uncinate process since a jagged or a free edge is required which can then be engaged into the shaver blade before it can be cut. The surgeon can create this jagged edge by using the reverse cutting forceps to cut the uncinate process at the junction of its vertical and the horizontal portion. The upper portion of the uncinate process can now be gently retracted forward using a blunt probe and its cut edge can then be worked upon with the blade of the microdebrider and the uncinectomy can be done in an upward direction all the way up to its attachment. This now enables the surgeon to work in the frontal recess area. Similarly, the inferior portion of the uncinate process can be worked upon with the microdebrider, with the blade window facing inferiorly and proceeding from anterior to posterior direction. This inferior portion of the uncinate can thus be completely removed. Removal of this lower portion will bring the maxillary ostium into view.

If necessary, it can be widened by using the shaver. Here again the mucosa of the posterior border of the ostium may be cut or punched with forceps to create a free edge which can then be enlarged by the microdebrider to the desired size without tearing away tissues from the surrounding areas. The microdebrider can also be used to complete the ethmoidectomy. After an uncinectomy, the bulla ethmodalis can be punctured with the blunt tip of the shaver blade and edges of the opening can be engaged in the blade to remove tissue superiorly and laterally to reach the skull base and lamina papyracea. Since the instrument remains parallel to the lamina papyracea and the base of the skull, the chance of damage to these structures is minimised. Once the anterior ethmoidal cells have been cleared and the ground lamella exposed, the soft tissue shaver can be used to puncture the lamella with its blunt tip and clear the posterior ethmoidal cells in a similar manner. One should be careful to avoid lateral dissection in the posterior ethmoids in view of the proximity of the optic nerve. Complete dissection of the anterior and posterior ethmoidal cells can thus be achieved without avulsing the adjacent mucosa.

If the surgeon now wishes to enter sphenoid sinus, he can continue to dissect with the shaver and use the blunt tip to enter the sphenoid sinus. Following removal of the posterior ethmoid cells, the surgeon can identify the posterior attachment of the superior turbinate, push the posterior edge of the superior turbinate medially with the blunt tip of the shaver; and identify the sphenoid ostium. The shaver blade can now be pushed into the sphenoid sinus through its anterior wall at the lower limit of the ostium. The shaver is then used to widen the ostium to gain access to the sinus. However, blindly pushing the blade into the depth of the sphenoid sinus and using it without proper visualisation should be avoided to prevent damage to vital structure on the lateral wall, viz., the optic nerve and internal carotid artery. In a significant percentage of patients, there may be a dehiscence of the optic canal. Therefore, any dissection within the sphenoid sinus without proper visualisation should certainly be avoided. If the natural ostium of the sphenoid sinus is not visualised as mentioned above, the tip of the shaver blade can be used to penetrate the anterior wall of the sphenoid sinus by approaching it through the nasal cavity following the nasal septum posteriorly and opening the anterior wall of the sinus a little above the roof of the posterior choana, and then widening the opening superiorly to reach the ostium.

The shaver blade can also be used to open agger nasi cells thus giving surgeon a good access to the frontal recess. Using a 45 or 70 degree endoscope and an angled shaver blade, the frontal recess area can be effectively cleared to open the frontal ostium in order to ventilate the frontal sinus.

It has been observed that failure after "adequate" endoscopic sinus surgery is often due to lateralisation of the middle turbinate, which adheres to the lateral wall of the cavity created, i.e. to the lamina papyracea, thus blocking drainage and ventilation of the sinuses. To prevent this, use of the spacers has been suggested. The technique described by Bolger, now termed as Bolgerisation, seems to offer a very simple solution to this problem. A raw area is created on the medial aspect of the middle turbinate at the adjacent part of the nasal septum. The turbinate can then be pushed against the septum using small pieces of packing material such as merocel. This leads to formation of adhesions between the medial surface of the middle turbinate and the nasal septum, thus ensuring that the middle turbinate does not lateralise, thus preserving the ventilation of the sinuses. This step of Bolgerisation is also easily achieved by using the microdebrider.

Microdebriders are used in resecting, granulomas and even tumours of the nose. Rhinosporidiosis, for example, is a problem with its propensity to recur at multiple sites due to seeding in the raw areas created during surgery. Its vascularity causes it to bleed profusely during surgery thus obscuring the surgeon's view. With microdebriders, the granuloma is quickly and effectively excised without any trauma to the surrounding mucosa, thus eliminating the possibility of seeding. Once the bulk of the granuloma is reduced, it is possible to identify the stalk of the lesion and its attachment. This is now grasped with a bipolar cautery forceps and removed after coagulating it, thus ensuring complete removal.

Similarly benign tumours and even inverted papillomas can be effectively tackled endoscopically, thanks to the microdebrider, which allows easy and safe debulking of the tumour till its base is clearly visualised and excised completely.

DISCUSSION

The introduction of powered instruments for FESS; especially the microdebrider has been a major breakthrough in the "Functional" aspect of FESS. The microdebrider offers many advantages, viz., precise and clean removal of pathological tissue without tearing away the adjacent mucosa, continuous suction during tissue removal ensuring unobstructed vision, and less bleeding. Since the surrounding mucosa is preserved, healing of the operated cavity is quicker, better, with less scarring and without synechiae. It has also been observed that the cavity appears much cleaner and the amount of cleaning and dressing required in the post-operative period is much less.

It was, however, felt that the microdebrider takes away the tactile information that the surgeon gets with the traditional forceps, i.e., with the forceps he is able to palpate the tissue before removing it. But this is not quite true since the shaver tip can be used initially for palpation to get the same tactile information that one would get with the traditional forceps. In addition to all the above-mentioned advantages, studies also showed that the tissue that was sucked inside retained its histological characteristics.

Despite all these advantages of the microdebrider, a few drawbacks do exist. Due to the tissue being sucked in along with the particles of bone and blood, the shaver blades and the suction system tend to get clogged. The simultaneous use of irrigation may help to a certain extent but clogging still remains a problem. A powerful suction is a big help and the surgeon can avoid clogging by periodically aspirating saline into the shaver system as he proceeds with the dissection. In event of blockage of the shaver blade, the surgeon would have to stop the surgery, detach the blade and clean it either by flushing it with a syringe or by using the stylet provided with the blades. One must also realise that the shaver is not a substitute for proper anatomical knowledge and surgical skill. There have been reports of inadvertent entry into the orbit with the shaver tip, instead of the maxillary ostium, and this can be dangerous as the blade could suck in the orbital fat and the orbital contents if the surgeon does not realise this mishap. The consequences would be disastrous.

To conclude, microdebriders (soft tissue shavers) have many advantages in FESS as compared to the traditional instruments. Less bleeding, less tissue trauma, better results, increased safety when properly used, are some of them. Microdebriders are still being modified and improved upon, and better shaver systems will definitely make their appearance in years to come.

FURTHER READING

1. Christmas DA, Krouse JH: Powered Instrumentation in Functional Endoscopic Sinus Surgery. I. Surgical Technique. Ear Nose Throat J 1996; 75:1.
2. Ferguson BJ, Di Biase PA, D'Amio F: Quantitative Analysis of Microdebriders used in Endoscopic Sinus Surgery. American Journal of Otolaryngology, 1999; 20(5), 294-97.
3. Gross WE, Soft-Tissue Shavers in Functional Endoscopic Sinus Surgery (Standard technique). Otolaryngologic Clinics of North America, Vol 30 (3), (Gross W.E, Becker D.G., eds.) W.B. Saunders Co., Philadelphia, 1997; 435-41.
4. Krouse JH, Christmas DA: Powered Instrumentation in Functional Endoscopic Sinus Surgery II. A comparative study. Ear, Nose, Throat J 1996; 75:1.
5. Mc Garry GN, Gana P, Adamson B: The Effect of Microdebriders on Tissue for Histological diagnosis, Clinical Otolaryngology 1997; 22 (4), 375-76.
6. Setliff RC, Parsons DS: The "Hummer": New Instrumentation for Functional Endoscopic Sinus Surgery. American Journal of Rhinology 1994; 8:6.
7. Setliff RC, III: New Concepts and the Use of Powered Instrumentation (the "Hummer") for Functional Endoscopic Sinus Surgery. In Advanced Endoscopic Sinus Surgery, 1st edition, (Stankiewicz J. A ed), Mosby Year Book Inc., Philadelphia, 1995; 161-70.

CHAPTER 6

Precancerous Status of Oral Lesions

Seoane J, Diz-Dios P., Garcia-Pola MJ, Varela P.

Since 1978, the WHO has defined "precancer" as precancerous lesion or precancerous condition. Both denote an increased risk of malignant transformation within the oral cavity but have slight clinical differences: A *precancerous lesion* is a morphologically altered tissue in which cancer is more likely to occur than on its apparently normal counterpart (leukoplakia, erythroplakia, actinic cheilosis). A *precancerous condition* is a generalised state associated with a significantly increased risk of cancer (lichen planus, discoid lupus erythematosus, immunosuppression, oral submucous fibrosis, xeroderma pigmentosum, sideropenic dysphagia, syphilis).

These terms imply a given area of the oral mucosa is statistically more probable to develop a cancer, although not every precancerous lesion or condition will end up as a neoplasm. This is why several authors suggest the utterance "potentially malignant lesions or conditions" as more accurate than precancerous lesion/condition.

Epidemiological distribution of these pathologies varies according to the geographical area because their pathogenia is determined by genetic factors, cultural habits and social and economical circumstances.

LEUKOPLAKIA

Oral leukoplakia has been redefined as "a predominantly white lesion of the oral mucosa that cannot be characterised as any other definable lesion; some oral leukoplakias will transform into cancer."

It is possible to establish a provisional diagnosis based on clinical criteria alone, but the final one has to be based on pathological criteria in order to identify the existence and degree of epithelial dysplasia and to be able to carry out a differential diagnosis with other lesions of similar clinical appearance. The term leukoplakia is exclusively clinical and has no histopathological implications.

A great number of studies show leukoplakias have a significant trend to malignant transformation, with ranges between 0; 13% and 6% and reaching values up to 14% in those cases where epithelial dysplasia can be proven. These marked differences amongst reports may well be due to the type of population studied, the length of follow-up periods or even to the treatment applied. In this sense, patients with oral leukoplakia have 5-fold risk of suffering from oral cancer than those without.

Two main questions about oral leukoplakia remain open for discussion: how to predict malignant transformation and when and how to treat them.

How to Identify Oral Leukoplakias that will Undergo Malignant Transformation?

It seems proven that several leukoplakias are precancerous, but the problem is how to identify them. Some clinical and pathological criteria can be used to describe leukoplakias with an increased risk of undergoing malignant transformation: these leukoplakias are found mainly on female patients elder than 50 with a lesion of unknown aetiology that has been in the mouth for a long period of time. This lesion typically has more than 1 cm of extension on the floor of the mouth and spreads to ventral surface and lateral borders of the tongue; the clinical appearance is non-homogeneous and *Candida albicans* can be found on its surface. A pathological study showing signs of epithelial dysplasia would complete the picture.

The term "epithelial dysplasia" describes chronic and progressive pathological changes in premalignant disorders of the oral mucosa. It is, thus, a pathological marker of malignant transformation. Dysplasia can be graded as *mild*, with very few dysplastic alterations of the lower stratum of the epithelium, as *moderate* dysplasia when 2 to 4 dysplastic characters can be detected in the lower 2/3 of the epithelium, and *severe* dysplasia when 5 or more dysplastic characters can be identified in the epithelium as a whole. In our experience, lack of polarity of basal cells, increased numbers of mitosis, cell polimorfism, thickened nucleoli and keratinisation of isolated cells or groups of cells are strongly associated to severe dysplasia.

There are no fully reliable markers able to identify leukoplakias that will transform into oral cancer. However, the establishment of correct clinical and pathological correlations, like presence of dysplasia and non-homogeneous clinical presentations (particularly erythroleukoplakia and proliferative verrucous leukoplakia) are the most faithful markers of malignant potential availabe at the moment. In the near future, research on genetic changes in oral leukoplakias may provide useful information too.

How to Diagnose and Treat Proliferative Verrucous Leukoplakias?

Proliferative verrucous leuloplakia is an entity of unknown aetiopathogenia, that somehow includes the whole spectrum between hyperkeratosis and squamous cell carcinoma. It is originally diagnosed as a leukoplakia without dysplastic signs that shows a verrucous and proliferative growth later on time. Characteristics of proliferative verrucous leukoplakias are progression throughout several years, persistence and slow, diffuse/multifocal growth.

Proliferative verrucous leukoplakia is a lesion with very bad prognosis due to its aggresive biological behaviour, high rate of recurrence, trend to malignant transformation and also because it is impossible to establish a correct diagnosis at early stages.

Case Report 1

A 65-year-old, non-smoker female who presents a non-dysplastic leukoplakia on buccal mucosa, that was treated surgically. Two years later the patient demands attention to a leukoplakia affecting alveolar mucosa, floor of the mouth and left buccal fold. The lesion is treated surgically and an abdominal skin graft used to restore the area. One year later, a leukoplakia of verrucous aspect is detected on the dorsum and right border of the tongue and right alveolar ridge (Fig. 6.1, Plate 1). Multiple incisional biopsies were obtained and the pathological diagnosis was verrucous hyperplasia with signs of moderate/severe dysplasia. Samples were negative for papillomaviruses and displayed a diploid DNA content. Treatment with CO_2 laser and chemoprophylaxis with etretinate was decided. After three years of follow-up, no signs of reccurrence could be recognised.

Biopsy for Oral Leukoplakias (Incisional vs Excisional Technique)

Different authors doubt about the need of biopsing homogeneous leukoplakias because of their lower risk of suffering transformation into cancer. Nevertheless, there is a wide consensus about the need of biopsing oral leukoplakias to establish a definite diagnosis and to allow categorisation of the lesion. The disagreement is now whether to take an incisional or an excisional biopsy.

Detractors of incisional biopsies argue this procedure is not fully diagnostic as there may be focal dysplastic changes within a predominantly normal epithelium, normal areas within a dysplastic epithelium and different degrees of dysplasia in different parts of the lesion. These facts would justify the need for serial removal of the lesion and analysis of every single section of it.

Although this method does not exclude the existence of focal dysplasia or carcinoma, we use incisional biopsies on a regular basis by means of a 4-5 mm punch. In non-homogeneous leukoplakias, we perform multiple biopsies directed by clinical criteria, like the existence of reddish areas, atrophic or erosive, indurated, thickened or symptomatic areas. Ancillary procedures (toluidine blue) are also employed to select the area where biopsy will be undertaken. All specimens should be sent independently to the pathologist along with a description of its location within the lesion.

When dealing with exophytic leukoplakia, incisional biopsy obtained by scalpel should include the margins of the lesion and be deep enough to obtain an area of connective tissue to determine the existence of an invasive pattern and to permit the establishment of a differential diagnosis with verrucous carcinoma.

The main disadvantage of complete removal of leukoplakias in primary care settings arises when the pathological diagnosis is cancer. In these situations some other therapies are normally needed and the permanence of part of the lesion may be helpful.

Case Report 2

A forty-year-old male patient with a lesion on the lateral border of the tongue diagnosed clinically as ulcerated leukoplakia that had appeared 1 month ago. An excisional biopsy (Fig. 6.2, Plate 1) was taken in a primary care setting and pathological analysis found an infiltrating carcinoma with positive surgical margins. (Fig. 6.3, Plate 1) shows the clinical image of the tongue at the moment the patient was seen at hospital. Where is the ulcer?

In order to avoid this problem, some authors suggest the complete removal of the lesion only in those leukoplakias whose size allows the removal of more than 1 cm of healthy tissue around the lesion to guarantee negative margins in case of cancer diagnosis.

When and How to Treat Oral Leukoplakias?

In order to use standardised systems to categorise oral leukoplakias, a classification and staging system has been proposed. This classification is based on the extent of the lesion, location, clinical aspect (homogeneous and non-homogeneous) and the presence and degree of epithelial dysplasia. This system has prognostic implications and permits optimisation of therapeutical decisions. The idea behind the treatment of oral leukoplakia should always be to prevent malignant transformation of the lesion. Thus, therapeutic decisions have to be based opon the knowledge of natural behaviour of the lesion, expectancies and morbidity of the different therapeutical options.

The first therapeutical approach consists on elimination of known risk factors for oral leukoplakia, particularly tobacco and local irritants. When dealing with nodular mouth-angle leukoplakias, an antifungal treatment with miconazol gel for two or three weeks is suggested. If no regression of the lesion is observed, a biopsy should be taken. At the same time, it would be recommeded to investigate levels of vitamin A, vitamin B_{12}, vitamin C, beta carotenes and folic acid, as well as to prescribe intake of fruits and vegetables. Persistence of risk factors would determine an unfavourable prognosis of the lesion in terms of recurrence of the original lesion, onset of a new leukoplakia or even the appearance of an oral carcinoma.

Non-dysplastic Leukoplakia. What to do?

Several authors suggest a wait-and-see attitude in patients with leukoplakias without dysplasia or with mild dysplasia. They propose periodical check-ups every 3 to 6 months and repeat biopsy in case of clinical signs of alarm but, as a rule, at least once within the first 3 years after initial diagnosis. On the other hand, our interventionist attitude is based both upon the knowledge of the risk of malignant transformation in non-dysplastic leukoplakias, and upon the fact that complete removal of leukoplakias has shown up to a 10% of malignancies in some series, even in leukoplakias considered as benign with a preoperative incisional biopsy. This attitude is specially justified in socially and economically weaker groups where it is particularly difficult to maintain and adequate follow-up programme, in leukoplakias extending over large areas, and in young patients with a large life expectation. In these situations, and having taken a biopsy, we vaporise the lesion with a 10 Watt CO_2 laser with an unfocused bean (Figs 6.4, 6.5, 6.6, Plate 1).

Dysplastic Leukoplakia. What to do?

Despite some authors consider there are no strong evidences about the advantages of interventionist attitudes over the non-interventionist ones in avoiding malignant transformation and albeit different reports describe the possibility of spontaneous regression of dysplastic leukoplakias, we keep a particularly interventionist attitude in these cases. Our attitude is based upon the experience that untreated oral leukoplakias display a more important trend to develop oral cancer and also on the fact that time itself is a prognostic factor for malignant transformation. Moreover, it has been proved surgical removal of the lesion has caused a decrease in the frequency of malignant transformation compared to untreated oral leukoplakias.

We would rather perform a surgical excision with scalpel or CO_2 laser, taking serial samples and carefully checking all surgical margins. Excision by means of a laser device allows pathological analysis of the sample using a 5 W focused laser as a cutting instrument. This permitting cell analysis for dysplasia and study of basal membrane although analysis of surgical margins is very difficult as they are carbonised 0.5 mm depth. Laser has the advantage over conventional scalpel—particularly in large leukoplakias—of reducing morbidity. Laser induces healing by second intention in 2 to 4 weeks; contraction and functional limitations are minimised. In our experience, percentages of recurrence agree with those published by other groups and range between 8 and 35%. These data justify a long post-operative follow-up and the eventual use of chemoprevention due to the risk of recurrences, new lesions or malignant transformation.

What can be Expected from Pharmacological Treatment in Oral Leukoplakia?

Several drugs have been used in the treatment of oral leukoplakias: 13-cis-retinoid acid or etretinate per os 1mg/kg body weight for two months, beta carotenes at a dosage between 30 and 90 mg/day for 3 to 6 months and vitamin E (alpha tocopherol), 400 U twice a day for 24 weeks with improvement reported in 40 to 70% of the cases. However, the main contribution of pharmacological treatment to the treatment of oral leukoplakias may well be the use of post-operative chemoprophylaxis. In this sense, fenretidine (4-HPR), 200 mg/day for 52 weeks has proved useful in the prevention of new leukoplakias and the use of topic retinoids (tretinoine) over the area treated with CO_2 laser, once healed, seems to be able to prevent recurrences while using the drug, although new clinical trials are needed with drugs of less adverse effects.

ERYTHROPLAKIA

The term erythroplakia denotes any red patch or spot on the mucosa, generally of velvety aspect whose clinical and pathologic features do not allow its classification as any other disorder. This lesion was originally described by Queirat in 1911 on the glans of a syphilitic patient, this is why the disorder was given the name "erythroplasie de Queirat". A great number of similar lesions have been described on vulva and oral mucosa since then. Nowadays, the association of erythroplakia and syphilis is considered an accidental finding.

The aetiology and pathogenesis of erythroplakia are unknown; but the same factors involved in oral cancer development might have also something to do with erythtoplakias. Thus, alcohol and tobacco are involved, as well as some other factors that contribute or favour the progression of the lesion, like nutritional defects or chronic irritation.

Erythroplakia does not seem to have a sexual predilection. Most cases are diagnosed at the sixth and seventh decades of life. This entity's real epidemiological incidence is not known; it is lower than leukoplakia's but the proportion of erythroplakias undergoing malignant transformation is much higher.

What are Erythroplakia's Clinical Features?

The term erythroplakia has only clinical implications. Whereas initially the surface of the lesion is smooth, after some time it may become invasive and develop a slightly thickened and indurated lesion. As a general rule, it is more frequent on buccal mucosa followed by tongue locations. If location of the lesion is analysed by sex, erythroplakias are more frequent on the floor of the mouth of men and on the tongue and oral mucosa of women. These lesions are relatively small and asymptomatic. Erythroplakia can be classified according to its clinical appearance as homogeneous erythroplakias, erythro-leukoplakias and speckled presentations (Figs 6.7 and 6.8, Plate 2).

What are the Prognosis and Treatment of Erythroplakias?

Erythroplakia has been considered an early sign of development of intraoral squamous cell carcinoma, either invasive or "*in situ*". This idea is backed by the finding that most erythroplakias are either a histopathological squamous cell carcinoma or show a severe epithelial dysplasia at the time of diagnosis.

The floor of the mouth is a high risk location for the lesion to suffer malignant transformation. It is widely accepted erythroplakias with severe dysplasia or "*in situ*" carcinoma without proper treatment will become invasive cancers. The period of time required to accomplish this transformation can be anything between months and several years. Thus, it is necessary to establish a rigorous follow-up programme for these patients and to avoid agents known to stimulate carcinogenesis. The first measure should be to eliminate those factors involved on its pathogenesis.

Incisional biopsy is a compulsory step to confirm clinical diagnosis and assess the degree of dysplasia. It is possible some focal carcinomatous changes can be missed by the technique, and therapeutical attitude will be conditioned by the results of the pathological study.

Dysplastic erythroplakias demand a particularly interventionist attitude, according to the criteria and procedures already described for leukoplakias. However, the need for serial surgical samples for histopathological study contraindicates vaporisation with CO_2 laser. Due to the possible existence of multiple dysplastic focci and its tendency to recurrence, a prolonged post-operative follow-up of the patient is mandatory.

ACTINIC CHEILOSIS

Actinic cheilosis is a diffuse, premalignant alteration of the lower lip vermilion that results from long-term or excessive exposure to the ultraviolet component of solar radiation. This entity is more frequent among male patients over 40 years-old whose profession involves open air activities and amongst immunocompromised patients or renal transplant recipients.

A light of a wavelength between 2900 and 3200 C would be able to induce an actinic cheilosis throughout successive inflammatory processes in mucosa and submucosa. These radiation would affect vascularisation and alter collagen and elastic fibres producing a phenomenon known as solar elastosis, with the appearance of a characteristic acellular, basophilic, amorphous substance in the subepithelial corion.

These lesions are easy to identify clinically. In the beginning, lower lip becomes atrophic, with a bright light greyish aspect and not quite elastic, like a paper sheet. As exposure to sunlight increases, keratosis and erosions arise and reach the angles of the mouth and the mucocutaneous junction blurring lip limits. Sometimes superimposed "leukoplakias" can be identified. However, ultraviolet radiation is not unanimously accepted as an aetiological factor in oral leukoplakias. Some other authors consider epithelium in actinic cheilosis suffer disorders in both maturation and keratinisation, accumulating keratin on the surface as patches simulating real leukoplakias.

Is Actinic Cheilosis a Real Precancerous Lesion?

Malignant potential of actinic cheilosis is not well defined, with percentages of malignant transformation ranging from 1 to 20%. The World Health Organisation considers this entity as a histologically precancerous lesion; this is an epidermal dysplasia due to actinic radiation. We consider this lesion fulfils the requirements to be considered clinically as precancerous, where often appear squamous cell carcinomas on non-treated cases and frequently show epithelial dysplasia with cytological atypia and increased mitotic activity. Carcinomas developing on actinic cheilosis usually are well differentiated with a non-aggressive biological behaviour, although metastasis arise in up to 13% of cases. Several hypotheses have been proposed to explain malignant transformation of actinic lesions; one of them suggests alteration of subepithelial connective tissue might affect the p54 tumour suppressor gene. Ultraviolet radiation would act, thus, as a carcinogenic agent.

When and How to Treat Actinic Cheilosis?

Despite the good results obtained, existing therapeutic techniques, like 5-fluorouracil, electrosurgery, cryosurgery, vermilionectomy with mucosal advancement and vaporisation or excision with CO_2 laser, have not fully solved the question about the best time for treatment and what technique to use.

Decision about treatment should be based on the information obtained from the previous incisional biopsy that should be directed to eroded or ulcerated areas, indurated or thickened zones or areas with keratosis in order to confirm the clinical diagnosis, to assess the degree of dysplasia and to discard the presence of a carcinoma within the lesion.

Most of the changes associated with actinic cheilosis will probably be unreversible and are related to the amount of ultraviolet radiation accumulated. However, we should stimulate preventive attitudes towards oral cancer, like the use of a protective lip balm containing para-amino-benzoic acid (PABA) or its derivatives. Substances protecting against radiation of a wavelength higher than 3200 A, like zinc oxide or titanium oxide can also be used.

Mild forms of actinic cheilosis can be treated by means of retinoic acid pomades or topic application of 5-fluoruracil that destroys and eliminates damaged epithelium but does not prevent the onset of new lesions. It can be applied either as a solution or as cream at 5% 3 or 4 times a day for two weeks or until erosion of the treated area is achieved.

In severe cases, and having excluded the possibility of a squamous cell carcinoma, we consider vermilionectomy as the first therapeutic option due to its good aesthetic and functional results, although the patient may experiment pain, paraesthesia and a feeling of tightness on the lip. As a surgical alternative, it is possible to vaporise the lesion with a 3 Watt CO_2 laser, unfocused and in continuous mode applied twice over the affected area. This technique improves postoperative period reducing oedema and haemorrhage and easing a rapid cicatrisation (Figs 6.9 and 6.10, Plate 2).

Case Report 3

A 67-year-old patient wihout relevant clinical history, smoker of 20 cigarettes per day for 47 years and alcohol abuser (1 lalcohol per day) demands attention to a lesion on his lower lip that had bled occasionally. Intraoral inspection shows 3 remaining teeth in very bad condition, a keratotic lesion on lip mucosa and a bluish atrophic lesion on the vermilion area; none of them tender to palpation. Two biopsies were taken, one from the intraoral lesion and the other from the lesion on lip semimucosa. The histopathological analysis of the first one revealed a hyper-keratosis that led to the diagnosis of leukoplakia. The second biopsy disclosed epithelial atrophy and dense connective tissue elastosis. The diagnosis was actinic cheilosis (Fig. 6.11, Plate 2).

ORAL LICHEN PLANUS AS A PRECANCEROUS CONDITION

Lichen planus is a chronic inflammatory mucocutaneous disease in which basal epithelial cells are damaged by a cell-mediated immune process, involving Langerhans cells, T-lymphocytes, and macrophages, not unlike that reported for allergic contact dermatitis and graft-vs-host disease.

Oral lichen planus slackens and worsens alternatively throughout its chronic evolution and might, eventually, suffer malignant transformation. Several studies have shown evolution of the disorder is independent from sex and initial clinical presentation of the lesion. The most important prognostic factor for healing seems to be the amount of inflammatory infiltrate in the corion; the higher the number or cells, the lower the probability of complete healing.

Can Oral Lichen Planus Undergo Malignant Transformation?

This is a controversial topic that is focusing the interest of the scientific community. There are important series where no cases changed into squamous cell carcinoma, but other series unveil percentages higher than those described for oropharyngeal cancer in common population. The main question here is: does oral lichen planus "per se" suffer malignant transformation? Three possible answers have been proposed:

- Lichen planus results on a more exposed epithelium external irritative factors, perhaps with carcinogenetic potential (Murti 1984, Pogrel 1983).
- Lichen planus suffers malignant transformation, as dysplastic signs can be seen in some lesions (De Jong 1984, Odykoya 1985).
- Those cases showing malignant transformation described in the literature are incorrectly diagnosed most of the times. These cases would be a new entity: lichenoid dysplasia, but not real oral lichen planus (Krutchoff 1985, Lovas 1989, Allen 1998).

The first hypothesis, probably the most widely accepted nowadays, considers oral lichen planus as a "premalignant condition". This idea is backed by the fact that it is the red type (atrophic-erosive) the one that suffers malignant transformation more frequently. This circumstance supports the theory that epithelium plays an important role. It has been proposed that lichen planus implies an increase in basal cells turnover that predisposes the development of a malignant clon in the presence of initiators or promoters of malignancies.

In India, the proportion of tobacco consumers among patients affected by lichen planus is high (93%) and Murti describes how the risk of suffering from oral cancer is increasing in comparison to those tobacco consumers without lichen planus. This led to the conclusion this pathology leaves epithelium more exposed to external irritative agents, like tobacco. It has been also considered that therapy with corticosteroids and immunosuppresors might have some relevance in the increased cancer risk in these patients due to the immunosuppresion these drugs induce. The role of herpes viruses in the disorder requires further investigation.

The high frequency of epithelial dysplasia (about 25%) found in oral lichen planus lesions has generated the hypothesis that this disorder is a precancerous lesion.

The third hypothesis about malignant transformation of oral lichen planus affirms that most of the cases published in scientific literature are diagnostic mistakes. In 1978, Krutchkoff et al, after reviewing all 222 cases of malignant transformation of oral lichen planus described until then, claimed only 15 cases could be really accepted. Eight of those 15 had had an unknown exposure to carcinogenetic agents and no information about this point was available for the other 7. This leads Krutchkoff to maintain his affirmation that malignant evolution of lichen planus is false. The other 207 cases were excluded because of laxity in diagnostic criteria or absence of data about a hypothetical exposure to carcinogenetic agents. However, Marder (1982), not so demanding, affirms there are 101 cases sufficiently documented where malignant transformation of an existing lichen planus had taken place.

Most of the "supposed malignant transformations" described in the literature do not fulfil the requirements for accepting the original diagnosis of lichen planus of the oral mucosa. In order to explain this phenomenon, the concept of lichenoid dysplasia has been developed. It can be defined as a lichenoid lesion with signs of dysplasia without, generally, degenerative signs in the basal stratum. Recent studies reinforce this idea at observing a low frequency of loss of heterozygosity (LOH) in oral lichen planus lesions and a high frequency of it in lichenoid dysplasia, suggesting they are different entities.

We believe there are enough evidences to support the affirmation the risk of cancer is increased in patients with oral lichen planus. In our experience, being a male, present atrophic-erosive types, being exposed to carcinogenetic agents and have a long period of evolution behave as risk factors (Fig. 6.12, Plate 2). At present times, the influence of hepatitis C virus is being discussed. However, more and more adequate epidemiological studies are needed to assess this increase in risk. It seems particularly important to consider the existence of lichen planus lesions that can be clinically misdiagnosed with leukoplakia or erythroplakia. Moreover, it must not be forgotten it is possible to find both lesions at the same time. Because of these facts, a pathological study of the lesion is mandatory to obtain a certain diagnosis and to determine the presence of epithelial dysplasia.

When and How to Treat Oral Lichen Planus?

It is widely accepted that reticular types of oral lichen planus do not require treatment and can be controlled with a suitable follow-up programme every 3 to 6 months. In plaquelike lichen planus, some authors have recommended the use of topic retinoids or etretinate. Our experience shows a good therapeutic response can be obtained by vaporisation with a 6-10 Watt CO_2 laser with unfocused beam (Figs 6.13, 6.14 and 6.15, Plate 3).

In atrophic-erosive types, treatment should be initiated using topic corticosteroids, as they are considered the most useful drugs in oral lichen planus treatment. Pomades in orabase of 0.1% triamcinolone acetonide, 0.05% clobetasol propionate, and 0.1% fluocinolone can be used three times per day. In very large lesions we suggest the use of aquous solutions of 0.1% triamcinolone three times per day. Systemic treatment with corticosteroids should be reserved for aggressive atrophic-erosive lesions that do not respond to topical treatment: prednisone at a dosage of 40-60 mg/day for a week and decrease dosage progressively. Clobetasol or betamethasone can be used as an alternative.

Severe types of oral lichen planus, refractory to conventional treatment can be treated by means of oral phototherapy (PUVA) or topic cyclosporine.

Oral PUVA therapy with low-dose UV-A was effective in treating oral lichen planus of various forms (erosive, atrophic, or reticular). Phototherapy (UVA) combined with psoralenes has showed an immunomodulating activity which makes it useful in the treatment of this disorder. At present time, and due to the lack of reports on the subject, there are not defined guidelines for treating oral lichen planus lesions. It is mandatory to exclude patients with hepatic or renal pathology or previous history of photoallergy from this procedure.

Case Report 4

ADG, female, 56-year-old, insulin-dependent diabetic, with an erosive oral lichen planus pathologically diagnosed 6 months ago, located on both buccal mucosas, tongue, gingiva, lower lip and hard palate. A topical treatment was established with 0.05% clobetasol dipropionate in orabase at a proportion of 1:1, three applications per day during two weeks. Once the treatment had finished, no changes in the lesions could be observed and the patient remained with her painful symptoms. Because of the inappropriateness of using systemic corticosteroids, the use of photochemotherapy was decided. As photosensitising agent 0.6 mg/body weight of 8-metoxipsoralene (oxsoralen) taken two hours before treatment. As irradiation source, a Waldman 200 unit (I: 9 mw/cm^2) was used. During treatment, an aluminium foil mask was made to protect the face of the patient. Treatment was started with an exposition of 45 seconds at 0.5 J/cm^2, increasing progressively in 15 seconds of treatment each session until a cumulative dosage of 35.9 J/cm^2 given in 20 sessions every second day. After the eleventh session, the patient refers disappearance of clinical symptoms, when the cumulative dosage was 12.3 J/cm^2. After treatment, erosive lesions had disappeared from buccal mucosa and dorsum of the tongue. Atrophic lesions remained and only a slight improvement was observed on reticular lesions on gingiva and hard palate. No changes were observed in urine and blood tests (Figs 6.16 and 6.17, Plate 3).

Topic cyclosporine could be indicated in refractory lichen planus. Mouthwashes with a 5 cc 10% cyclosporine in olive oil for five minutes, three times per day during 8 weeks have proved effective for the treatment of oral lichen planus, particularly in severe and erosive forms. However, clinical trials failed to identify better therapeutical results when compared to topic corticosteroids.

DISCOID LUPUS ERYTHEMATOSUS AS A PRECANCEROUS CONDITION

Lupus erythematosus is a chronic disorder affecting connective tisue, that evolves in outbreaks, caused by an alteration of the immune system balance. Its aetiopathogenia is not well understood, but genetic (HLA B-7 y B-8, CW-7, Dr-2, DR-3 y DQ W-1), and neuroendocrine factors have been suggested, as well as precipitating agents like drugs, ultraviolet radiations and transmittable agents. Oral lupus erythematosus is rare, and its incidence ranges from 10 to 25% for discoid forms and from 30 to 50% for disseminated lupus erythematosus. Clinical diagnosis is complicated by the existence of non-discoid or atypical discoid oral lesions. However, when typical discoid oral lesions are present, diagnosis is suggested by the identification of an atrophic central area surrounded by keratotic papules located preferably on buccal mucosa. Diagnosis of certainty is based upon clinical, histopathological and immunopathological criteria.

What is Discoid Lupus' Potential for Malignant Transformation? Where should we Look?

Classically, malignant transformation of discoid lupus erythematosus was close to 30%, but it must be born in mind that these cases were treated with radiotherapy. Nowadays, this rate is about 0.2%. Special attention should be paid to the atrophic epithelium of lower lip's vermilion where malignant transformation is more likely to occur. Men are more propense than women to develop a cancer on this area. This could be due to the higher propensity of males to suffer lip cancer, to sun exposure or even to the amount of time the lesion has to progress. In our experience it is of utmost importance not to mistake typical features of lupus on the lip, like asymmetrical thickening caused by inflammatory infiltrate or like skin invasion by semimucosal lesion with malignant transformations.

Case Report 5

A 21-year-old woman demands attention to a pain in her TMJ and to repeating subluxations of this joint. Intraoral inspection shows an enantema of 1 cm diameter. Palpation permits good delimitation of this gummy lesion (Fig. 6.18, Plate 3). The lesion is biopsied and pathological study describes epithelial atrophy, a marked perivascular inflammatory infiltrate, connective tissue oedema and hydropic degeneration of the basal layer. Considering these findings, immunofluorescence tests were made to confirm the diagnosis of lupus erythematosus. A systemic study of the patient was made and haemolytic anaemia, urine proteins higher than 0.5 gm/day and antinuclear antibodies were the most interesting findings.

IMMUNOSUPPRESSION

It has been suggested cell immunity plays a main role in the genesis of premalignant lesions and in their progression towards cancer. As a consequence, severe immunodepressed patients are particularly at risk of oral cancer. Immunossuppresion itself favours the onset of other fatal diseases, usually of infectious origin, that cause death of these patients before intraoral neoplasms occur. However, there are patients with immunological disorders, as transplant recipients and those infected by human immunodeficiency virus (HIV), whose survival has noticeably increased in recent years and, as a result, so has the risk of developing precancerous lesions and oral cancer.

Transplant Recipients

These patients have shown an important prevalence of premalignant cutaneous lesions, reaching up to 19% in some series of renal transplant patients. A frequent feature of these lesions is hyperkeratosis, being its usual clinical presentation verrucous lesions, keratotic leukoplakias and keratoacanthomas. A great percentage of these lesions showed several types of *Human papillomaviruses*. This fact lead to the conclusion that this micro-organism may be entangled on initial phases of cancer genesis, acting presumably as a tumour-promotive agent that favours cell proliferation. In transplant-recipient patients, predisposing factors of premalignant lesions, like age and actinic radiation should also be taken into account.

Management

Although appearance of precancerous lesions on stomatological areas is rare, kidney transplant receivers seem to be particularly affected by neoplasms of the lip. Thus, avoidance of prolonged sun exposure is recommended particularly for adult and aged patients. Every intraoral or perioral suspicious lesion should be studied pathologically, particularly those of keratotic aspect. Antibiotic prophylaxis is mandatory, and haematological status should be investigated before biopsy (erythrocytes, leukocytes with differential and blood-plaques).

Case Report 6

A twenty-two-year-old male who had received a bone marrow transplant five years ago presented an asymptomatic white lesion on hard palate, clinically and pathologically compatible with

Plate 1

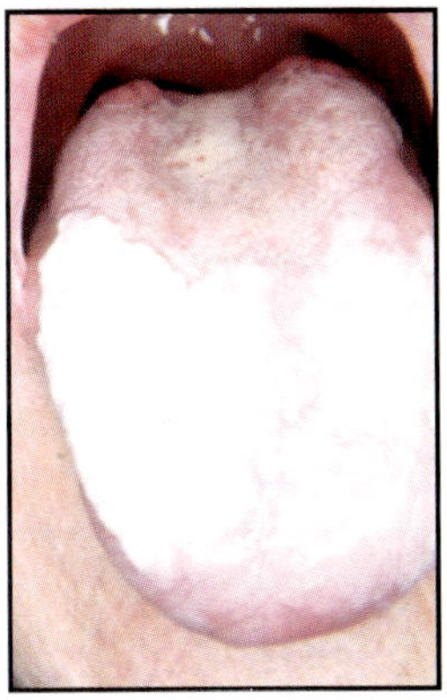

Fig. 6.1: Verrucous leukoplakia on the dorsum of the tongue

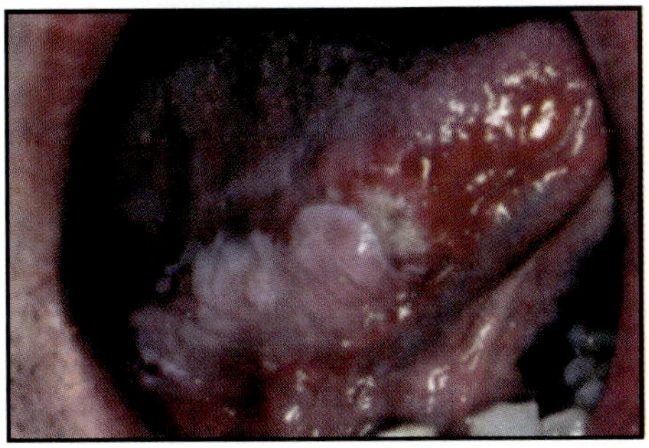

Fig. 6.2: Ulcerated leukoplakia

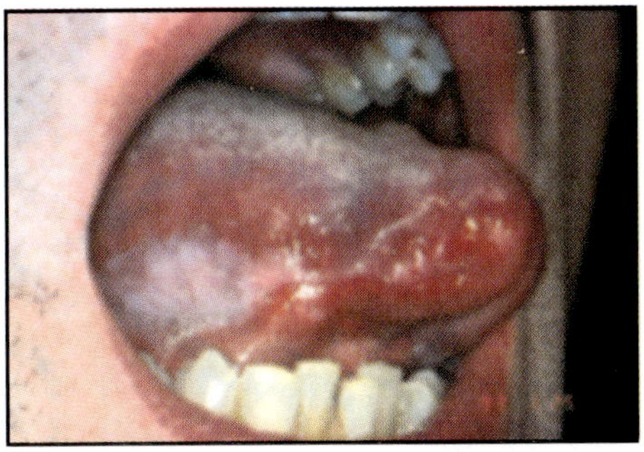

Fig. 6.3: Residual leukoplakia after excisional biopsy of the ulcer

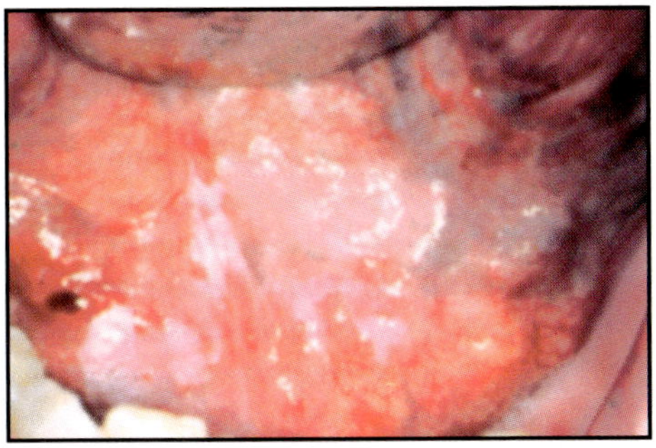

Fig. 6.4: Homogeneus leukoplakia on the floor of the mouth

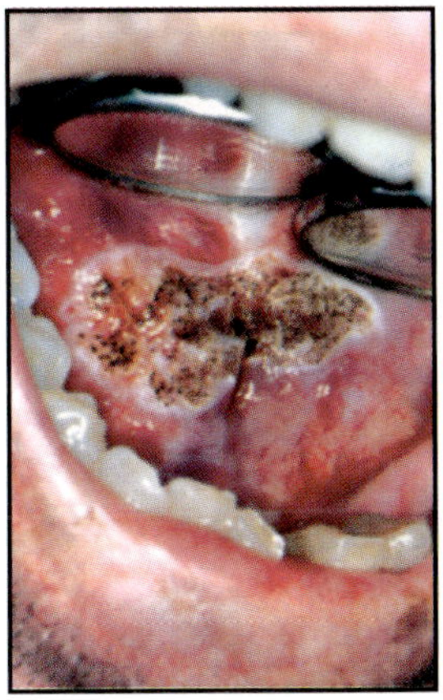

Fig. 6.5: Postoperatory view after laser vaporisation

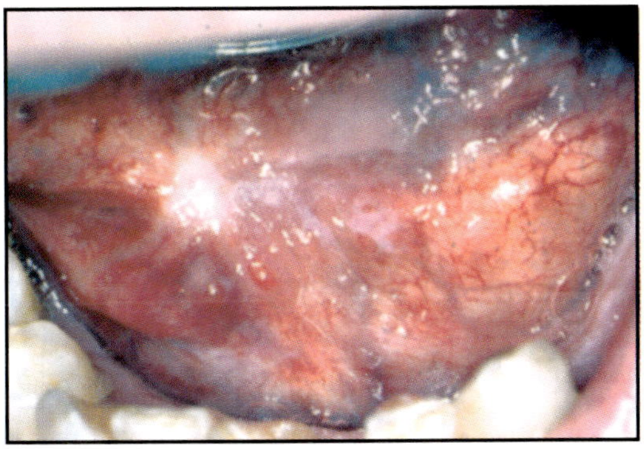

Fig. 6.6: Final clinical aspect (1 month later)

Plate 2

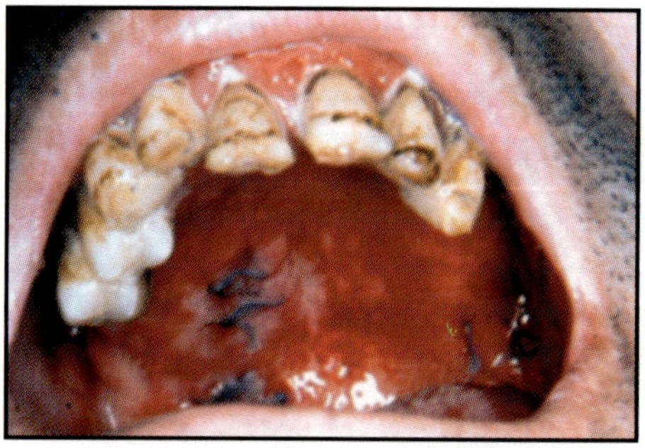

Fig. 6.7: Homogeneus erythroplakia

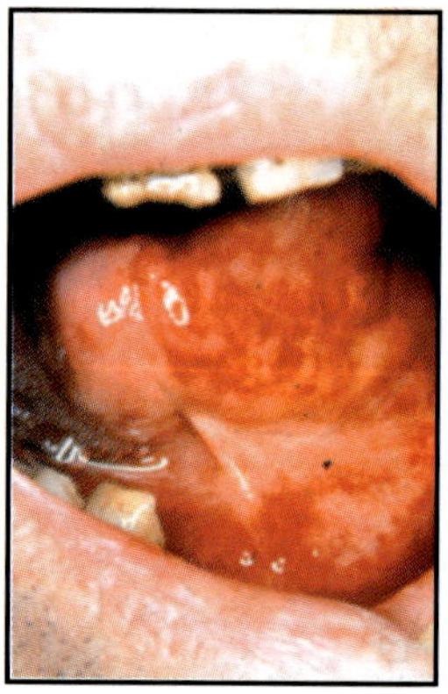

Fig. 6.8: Erythroplakia on the tongue and floor of the mouth

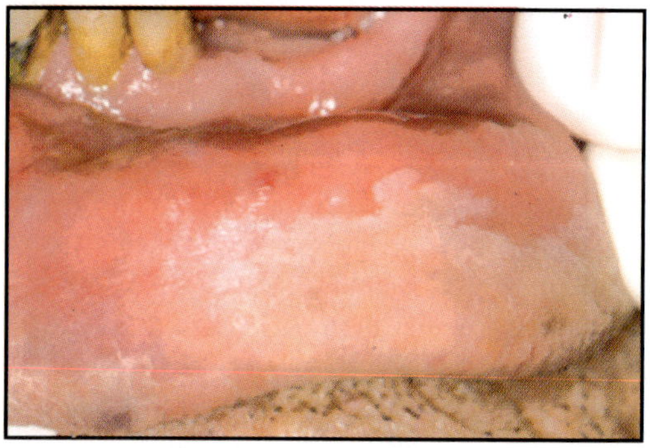

Fig. 6.9: Actinic cheilosis

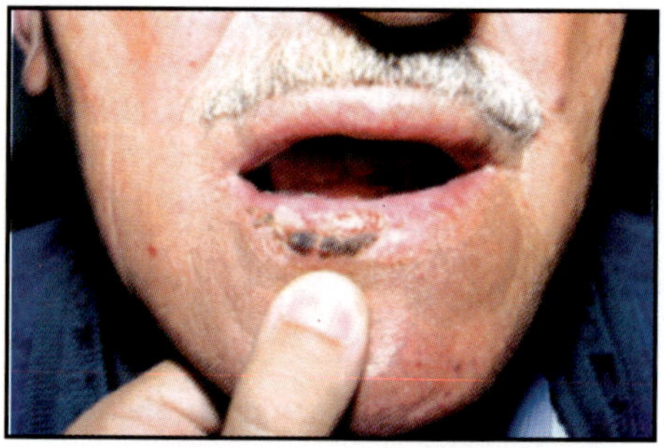

Fig. 6.10: Actinic cheilosis after laser vaporisation

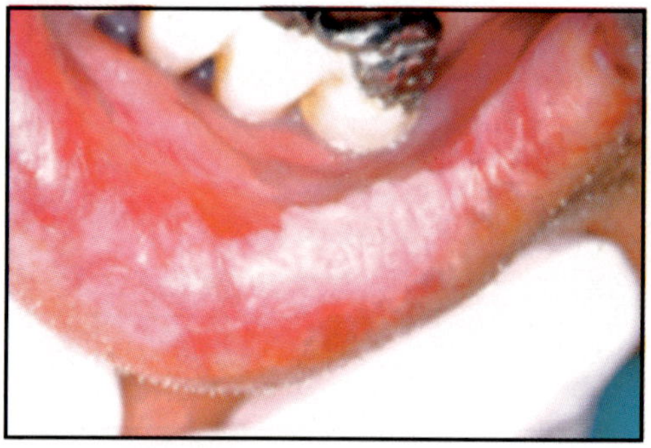

Fig. 6.11: Keratotic actinic cheilosis

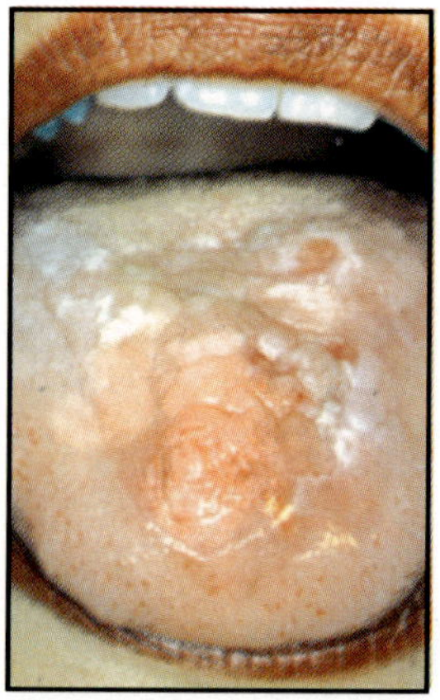

Fig. 6.12: Squamous cell carcinoma located on a previous atrophic—erosive lichen

Plate 3

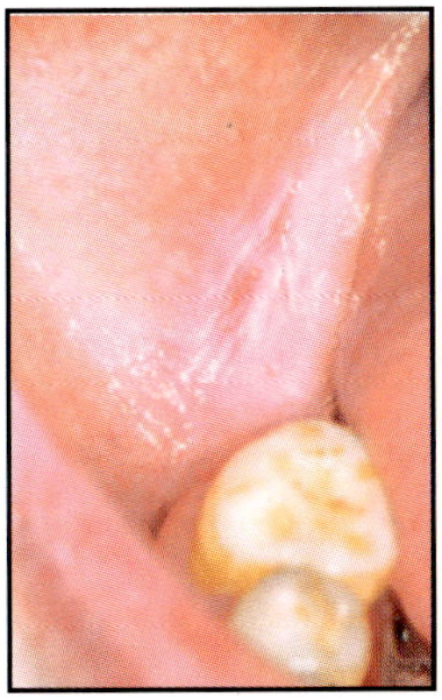

Fig. 6.13: Residual plaquelike lichen after topic cyclosporine

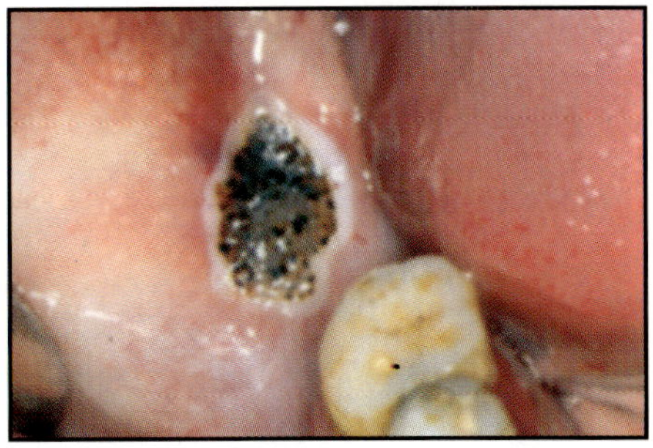

Fig. 6.14: Postoperatory view after laser vaporisation

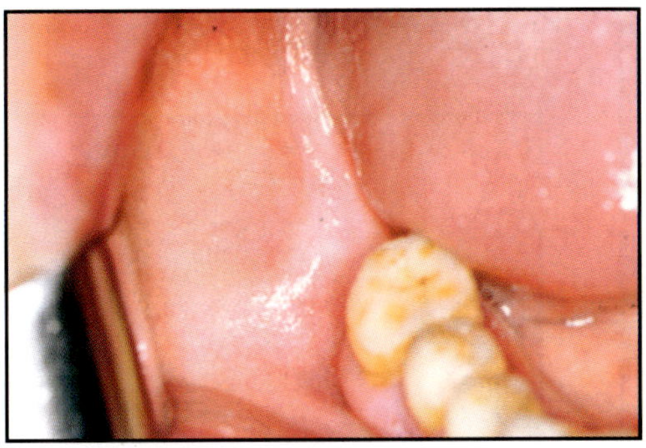

Fig. 6.15: Final clinical aspect (1 month later)

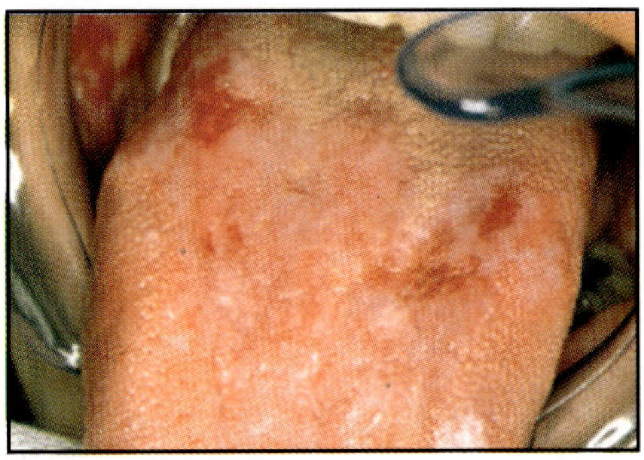

Fig. 6.16: Severe atrophic-erosive lichen on the dorsum of the tongue

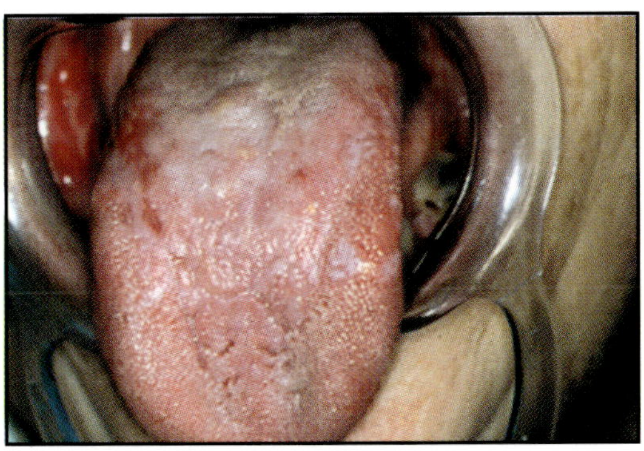

Fig. 6.17: Lesions resolution after PUVA treatment

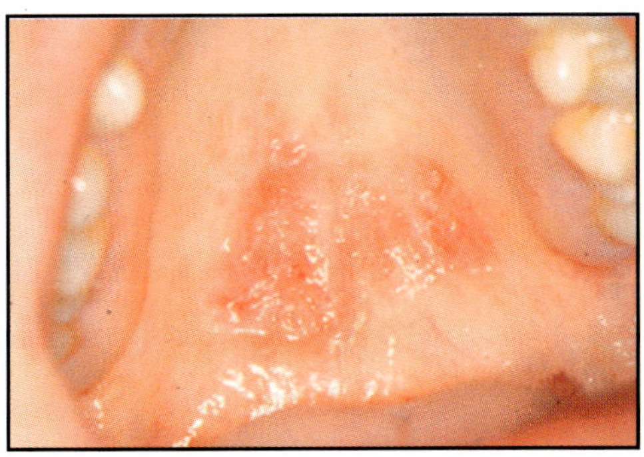

Fig. 6.18: Erythematous lupus on the hard palate

Plate 4

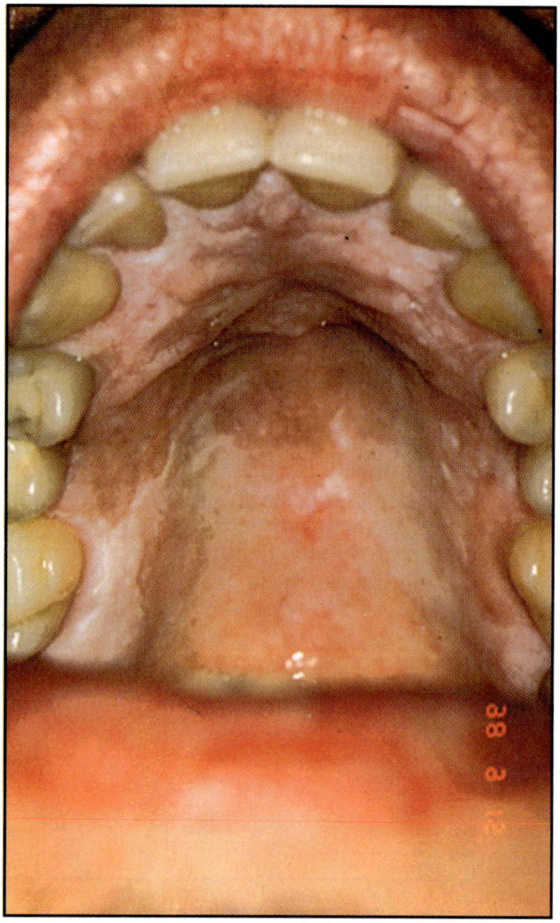

Fig. 6.19: Keratotic lesion on the palate in a bone marrow transplant patient

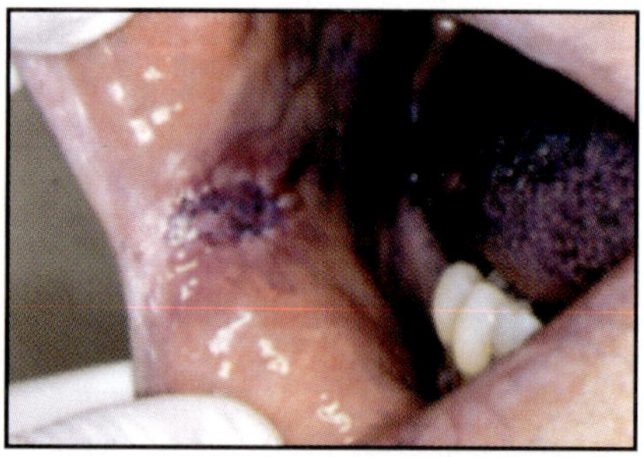

Fig. 6.20: Non-homogeneus retrocomisural Candida-leukoplakia stained with toluidine blue

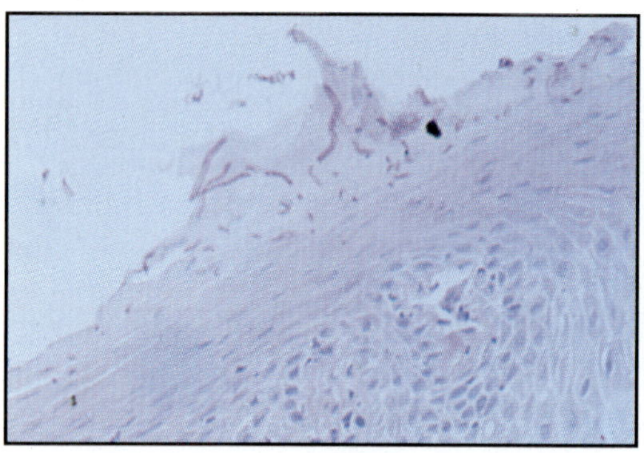

Fig. 6.21: Histopathologycal study of a non-homogeneus Candida-leukoplakia (H and E × 40)

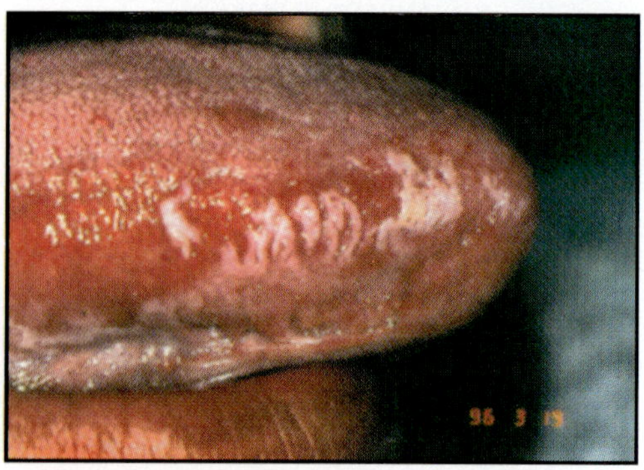

Fig. 6.22: Hairy leukoplakia

Plate 5

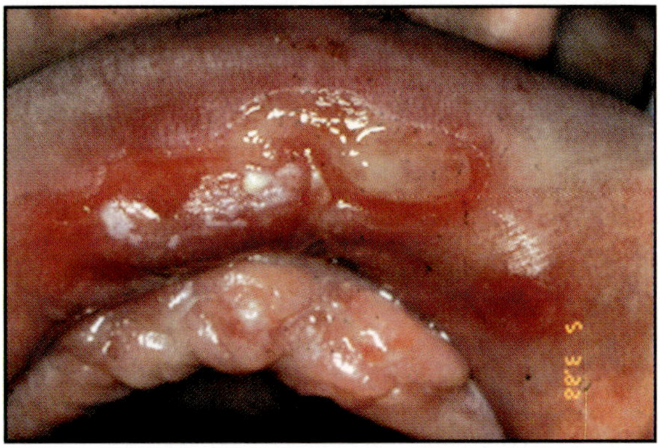

Fig. 6.23: Vesicular and erosive oral presentation of secondary syphilis

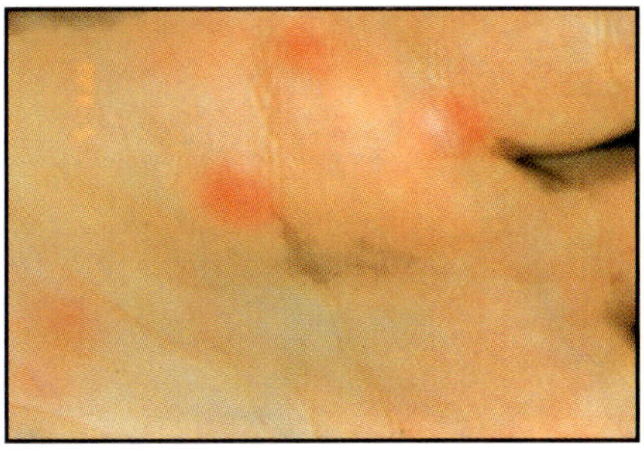

Fig. 6.24: Skin syphilides

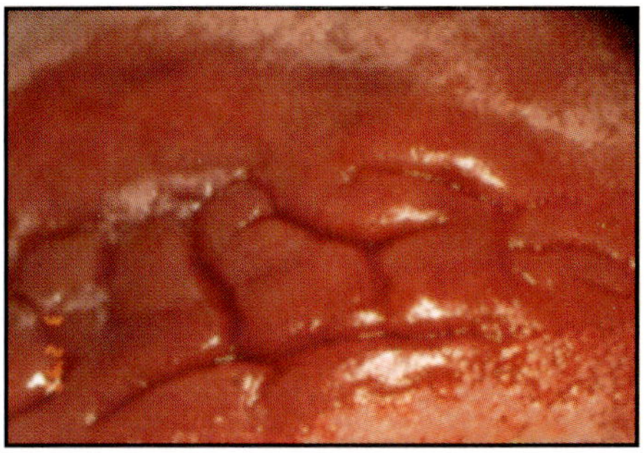

Fig. 6.25: Atrophic and interstitial glossitis in the same patient

keratotic leukoplakia several months after transplantation (Fig. 6.19, Plate 4). Despite its homogeneous aspect, the patient was trained in self-exploration techniques and a follow-up programme at his GDP's was established.

HIV-positive Patients

In the beginning, squamous cell carcinoma was considered a frequent disorder in HIV-positive patients, but results obtained from large series in Italy and the USA failed to corroborate this relationship. Most cases in the literature began as leukoplakias or erythroplakias on the posterior third of the tongue, floor of the mouth, tonsilar region or soft palate that evolved to induration or ulceration. These tumours have been related to the interaction of several factors (immune dysfunction, viruses and cell proliferative index) along with known risk factors (alcohol, tobacco, previous radiotherapy) on areas with high potential of malignant transformation.

It is widely accepted HIV-positive patients neither experience a higher incidence of these lesions nor a higher percentage of malignant transformations than HIV-negative ones. There are no HIV-infection pathognomonic precancerous lesions and it is not possible to predict whether better survival rates of HIV patients will involve an increase in the incidence of intraoral neoplasms.

Infectious disorders are common in HIV-patients due to their progressive immuno-compromise. Two white lesions related to infective agents can be identified in these patients, and both of them could be grouped under the wide definition of leukoplakia: *Hairy leukoplakia*, related to recurrent infections by Epstein-Barr virus, can be typically found on lateral borders of the tongue. It is a benign, asymptomatic lesion that does not undergo malignant transformation. Usually no treatment is required. *Candidal leukoplakia*, or hyperplastic candidiasis can be preferably found on buccal mucosa, and it is the clinical expression of a chronic infection by *Candida spp*. Its response to antifungal therapy is equivocal. Some reports describe this lesion as potentially malignant (Figs 6.20 and 6.21, Plate 4).

Management

When a lesion suggestive of candidal leukoplakia is seen, presence of *Candida spp* should be confirmed by taking a smear. If diagnosis is confirmed, systemic treatment should be established. We recommend fluconazole (100-200 mg/day) or itraconazole (200 mg/day) for two weeks. After treatment, remnant suspicious lesions should be biopsied (preferably by excisional technique) avoiding transmission of the infection. Before biopsy procedures, a blood test including red cells, leukocytes with differential, blood-plaques, hepatic enzymes and coagulation analysis should be performed.

Case Report 7

A thirty-five-year-old, HIV-positive male with a white, asymptomatic lesion on lateral borders of the tongue, clinically and pathologically compatible with hairy leukoplakia. No follow-up programme is established as the lesion will not undergo malignant transformation (Fig. 6.22, Plate 4).

ORAL SUBMUCOUS FIBROSIS

First described by Pindborg in 1964, it is a precancerous condition of insidious evolution that can affect all mucosal areas within the oropharynx. Its main feature is loss of elasticity in the affected mucosa causing severe functional limitations. Histologically, it is no uncommon to find signs of epithelial dysplasia that would account for its high frequency of malignant transformation.

This disorder is more frequent in South East Asia, particularly in India and, to a lesser extent, in Sri Lanka, Malaysia, Nepal, Thailand, Pakistan and China. It is rare in Western countries, and the cases observed in the UK and Australia were immigrants of Indian origin. It is more frequent about the age of 40, and prevalence is similar in males and females.

Its origin has been related to areca nut chewing although a multifactorial aetiology has also been proposed. Nutritional errors (vitamin B deficiency) and immunological disorders associated to chronic irritation (spicy foods, tobacco, etc.) would act upon a status of hypersensitivity to spicy food or to betel nut chewing inducing an atrophy that would make oral mucosa more permeable to certain carcinogenetic agents.

The onset of the disease is a burning sensation in the oral mucosa accompanied by a dysgeusia demonstrable by electrogustometry in 46% of the cases, although patients do not refer subjective loss of taste. Mucosa loses its elasticity and generally symmetric fibrous bands are formed in cheeks, lips, gingiva, tonsil arch and floor of the mouth preventing tongue protrusion and difficulty in swallowing and blowing actions. Trismus, otalgia and deafness are other sequela of this disorder. Blisters, ulcers and intense mucous paleness with a typical "grained marble" aspect accompanied by intense tongue depapillation can be seen in some cases. Oral cancer coexists with submucous fibrosis in 40-50% of the cases reported in India.

Management

Pharmacological treatment is exclusively palliative and consists of submucous administration of an aquous extract of human placenta alone or associated with corticosteroids or hyaluronidase, vitamin A or topic corticosteroids and iron *per os*. Preventive counselling is extraordinarily relevant: correct nutritional errors and avoid chronic irritant factors, as tobacco, spicy food and betel nut consumption. Multiple biopsies must be performed, as squamous cell carcinoma has been found histologically in 5 to 6% of submucous fibrosis cases without clinical signs of carcinoma.

XERODERMA PIGMENTOSUM

Xeroderma pigmentosum is a rare autosomal recessive dermatosis, linking defective DNA repair with clinical abnormalities and neoplasm. The disease is often fatal before age of ten, but older patients have been described, with predominant skin, ophthalmic and neurologic involvement. Ultraviolet light-induced damage to the skin begins early and results in multiple tumours, especially in sun-exposed areas of the head and neck. Primary squamous cell carcinomas of the lip and anterior third of the tongue occur with increased frequency. Basal cell carcinomas and melanomas are not uncommon.

Management

Dentists and otorhinolaryngologists have to be aware of xeroderma pigmentosum oral and perioral manifestations. Dentists must avoid ultraviolet light-curing units in these patients.

SIDEROPENIC DYSPHAGIA

Sideropenic dysphagia is a precancerous condition characterised by an essential hypochromic microcytic anaemia named Kalznelson's cloroanaemia or ferropenic dysphagia. It is also known as Plummer-Vinson syndrome or Paterson-Brown-Kelly syndrome. Waldeström, who introduced the term "sideropenia" suggested anemia was not necessary for the disease to appear.

This disorder is seen mainly in women (only 4% of the patients are male) between the ages of 30 and 50. Its prevalence is higher in Scandinavian countries (Sweden), central Europe and among anglo-saxon populations in USA and UK. Sideropenic dysphagia is hard to find in black individuals and is an exceptional finding in areas like Polinesia, where only one case has been described.

Clinical features of this disease are tiredness, fatigue, dry mouth, angular cheilitis, early loss of teeth, diffitulty to swallow and to wear removable dentures, palenes of skin and mucosa, brittle hair, koilonychia, epigastric pain, tachycardia and effort dyspneoa. About 80% of patients suffer achlorhydria and seldom histamine-resistant total aquilia.

Though this syndrome is caused by iron deficiency, there are other coadjuvant factors like diet poor on vitamins and animal proteins, self-immune phenomena (antibodies against gastric mucosa) and previous gastric lesions.

Although it has been described dysphagia is due to oesophageal spasms, some authors impute it to the presence of membranes in the upper oesophageal tract whose origin could be related to a deprivation oesophagitis with atrophy and hyperkeratinisation of the mucosa that organises as fibrous bands in late stages that turn the existing functional dysphagia into an obstructive one. An Indian report by Khosla SN disclosed 13% of patients suffering from iron-deficiency anaemia presented dysphagia and only 4% of them had membranes; none of the patients with other types of anaemia nor any of the controls showed either dysphagia or membranes. Radiological studies with contrast materials detected oesophageal membranes in 59% of the patients with dysphagia. There can be dysphagia for solid elements in the presence of small-sized membranes or even in the absence of mechanical stenosis. Dysphagia can suddenly disappear once iron supplementation therapy has begun even though large membranes remain.

Single or multiple leukoplakias or carcinomatous lesions (squamous cell carcinomas) can develop on these atrophic areas within mucosa, particularly on the limit between hypopharynx and upper part of the oesophagus, close to the posterior part of the cricoid cartilage.

Management of a Sideropenic Dysphagia Patient

Treatment with ferrous sulphate is the only effective one, and is able to eliminate dysphagia and to diminish membranes size. Its efficacy depends upon how early treatment is started, although transformation of a Paterson-Brown-Kelly syndrome into a carcinoma can happen several years after a successful treatment with iron has been completed. Prevalence of sideropenic dysphagia has diminished in recent years due to diet improvements and also to treatment with inorganic iron salts. Early diagnosis is of utmost importance to prevent hypopharynx cancer. A dysphagia resistant to 14 days of conventional therapy requires a detailed exploration of larynx, hypopharynx and oesophagus.

SYPHILIS

Epidemiological studies have shown that oral cancer incidence and specifically cancer of the tongue, was significantly elevated among people with antecedent of syphilis infection. Although some authors do not consider tertiary syphilis a significant factor in oral cancer, it is generally accepted that an inadequately treated or untreated syphilitic leukoplakia may undergo malignant transformation.

Macular and papular syphilides, mucous patches and condylomata lata, are the most common manifestations of secondary syphilis. The main lesions related to late oral syphilis are gumma (which often involves the palate), atrophic and interstitial glossitis (both may lead to the development of leukoplakia and squamous cell carcinoma).

Oral Syphilis and HIV Infection

Oral involvement in patients with secondary or tertiary syphilis was very unusual in Western Europe until HIV pandemic disease began. Immune defects associated with HIV infection may lead to an altered clinical presentation, atypical serological courses and a more aggressive course ("malignant syphilis" is 60 times more frequent than in historic syphilis series) in patients infected with *Treponema pallidum*. Neurosyphilis is found in one sixth of those with active syphilis and, therefore, lumbar puncture should be considered as routine. Ulceronodular variety, white plaques or papules, erythematous and serpentine patches have been described in the oral cavity of HIV-infected patients. In consequence, syphilis should be included in the differential diagnosis of uncommon oral lesions in HIV-infected patients. In a study performed in Cleveland (USA), syphilis antibodies were detected in 8% of patients with neoplasms of the tongue. So serological investigations should be warranted in the initial assessment of all patients with oral cancer.

Case Report 8

A thirty-two-year-old woman with moderately painful multiple lesions in oral cavity that had appeared 3 weeks ago, and a small pruriginous papula on the skin. The definitive diagnosis was syphilis, and serological test for HIV infection also resulted positive (Figs 6.23, 6.24 and 6.25, Plate 5).

ORAL PRECANCER RELATED TO REVERSE SMOKING

The habit of reverse smoking (e.g., smoking with the lighted end inside the mouth) is practised in various parts of the world, especially in South East Asia (India). This habit is very uncommon in western countries. The first case of reverse smoking in the Netherlands was reported in 1987. Frequency of reverse smoking is higher in females than in males.

In a community-based, cross-sectional study carried out in the Philippines, the majority (over 95 per cent) of reverse smokers exhibited palatal mucosal changes including leukoplakia, mucosal thickening, fissuring, pigmentation, nodularity, erythema and ulceration. In comparison, only 26 per cent of conventional smokers exhibited macroscopic mucosal changes. Strong link between *bidi* smoking and central papillary atrophy of the tongue has also been demonstrated in rural Indian populations.

Palatal keratosis is very stable, whereas red areas change into nonpigmented areas. Epithelial dysplasia is common, the highest rate being in the red areas. Educational attainment, use of non-filtered cigarettes and duration of smoking have been related to oral lesions development. An inverse relationship between the incidence of palatal lesions and vitamin A intake has also been described.

Management

Health professional's main responsibilty is to insist in the need of habit cessation, as regression of lesions is high (87%) among those who stop their smoking habit. Educational programmes should be adapted to the idiosyncrasy of the region as in some countries (i.e. India) there are two subpopulations of smokers: the educated, white collar cigarette smokers, might respond to measures that make non-smoking fashionable. Less educated, low income people who smoke *bidi* or *chutta* may need strategies aimed at socioeconomic improvement.

A follow-up programme of palatal keratosis should be established, and taking biopsies only from suspicious lesions (heterogeneous, erosive, etc). All lesions displaying red areas should be biopsied in order to discard epithelial dysplasia.

FURTHER READING

Leukoplakia

1. Aguado A, Valbuena L, Seoane J, Vázquez J, Asenjo JA. Leucoplasia Verrucosa Proliferativa(LVP). Un comportamiento biológico infrecuente. Rev Esp Cirug Oral y Maxilofac 1995; 17:109-12.
2. Axéll T, Pindborg JJ, Smith CJ, van der Waal I. And a International collaborative Group on Oral White Lesions, Oral white lesions with special reference to precancerous and tobacco-related lesions:conclusions of an international symposium held in Uppsala, Sweden, May 18-21, 1994. J Oral Pathol Med. 1996; 25:49-54.
3. Brugère J, Szpirglas H. Lésions précancereuses des voies aero-digestives supérieures. Actualités de carcinologie cervico-facial Ed. MASSON Paris 1994.
4. Chiesa F, Sala L, Costa L, et al. Excision of oral leukoplakia by CO_2 laser on an out-patient basis: a useful procedure for prevention and early detection of oral carcinomas. Tumori, 1986; 72:307-12.
5. Chiesa F, Tratadi N, Sala L, et al. Follow-up of oral leukoplakia after carbon dioxide laser surgery. Arch Otolaryngol Head and Neck Surg 1990; 116:177-80.
6. Dunsche A, Fleiner B, Terheyden H, Hoffmeister B. Use of Carbon Dioxide Laser in the Therapy of Benign Oral Soft-Tissue Lesions. Rudert H, Werner JA(eds): Lasers in Otorhinolaryngoloy, and in Head and Neck Surgery. Adv Otorhinolaryngol. Basel, Karger, 1995, vol 49, pp136-39.
7. Fleiner B, Plath Thomas. Histological evaluation of leukoplakia following CO_2 Laser Excision. A clinical and experimental study. Rudert H, Werner JA(eds): Lasers in Otorhinolaryngology, and in Head and Neck Surgery. Adv Otorhinolaryngol. Basel, Karger, 1995, vol 49, pp125-29.
8. Gupta PC, Mehta FS, Daftary DK, et al. Incidence rates of oral cancer and natural history of oral precancerous lesions in a 10-year follow-up study of Indian villagers. Community Dental and Oral Epidemiology 1980; 8:287-333.
9. Gupta PC, Murti PR, Bhonsle RB, Metha FS, Pindborg JJ. Effect of cessation of tobacco use on the incidence of oral mucosa lesions in a 10-yr follow-up study of 12,212 users. Oral Diseases 1995; 1:54-58.
10. Hansen LS, Olson JA, Silverman S. Proliferative verrucous leukoplakia : A long-term study of 30 patients. Oral Surg Oral Med Oral Pathol 1985; 60:285-89.
11. Lamey PJ. Management options in potentially malignant and malignant oral epithelial lesions. Community Dental Health 1993; 10:53-62.
12. Lumerman H, Freedman P, Kerpel S. Oral epithelial dysplasia and the development of invasive squamous cell carcinoma. Oral Surg Oral Med Oral Pathol 1995; 79:321-29.
13. Seoane J, Bascones A, Ortiz S, Asenjo JA. Leucoplasia bucal:estudio histopatológico de 55 casos. Medicina Oral 1996; 2:6-14.
14. Silverman S, Gorsky M, Lozada F. Oral leukoplakia and malignant transformation. A follow-up study of 257 patients. Cancer 1984; 53:563-68.
15. Tratadi N, Grigolat R, Calabrese L. et al. Oral Leukoplakias: to Treat or Not? Oral Oncol 1997; 33:317-21.
16. Van der Waal I, Schepman KP, van der Meij EH, Smeele LE. Oral Leukoplakia : a clinicopathological review. Oral Oncol 1997; 33:291-301.

Erythroplakia

17. Bagàn Sebastián JV. Medicina oral. Lesiones y estados precancerosos. In : Bagàn Sebastiàn JV. Medicina oral. Barcelona: Masson, 1995: 166-74.
18. Bengel W, Veltman G. Differential diagnosis of diseases of the oral mucosa. Chicago: Quintessence Books, 1989.
19. Brightman V. Lesiones rojas y blancas de la mucosa bucal. In : Lynch MA: Medicina Bucal de Burket. Diagnòstico y tratamiento. Mèxico DF: Nueva Editorial Interamericana, 1986: 202-82.
20. Mashberg A. Erythroplasia: the earliest sign of asymptomatic oral cancer. J Am Dent Assoc 1978; 96: 615-20.
21. Precàncer y càncer oral. Algunos datos y estadìsticas. Pindborg JJ y col. Europa contra el càncer. Ilustre Consejo General de Colegios de Odontòlogos y Estomatòlogos. Madrid: SYSTEM BCN, SL, 1995.
22. Schwartz RA, Stoll HL. Èpithelial precancerous lesions. In : Fitzpatrich Th y cols. 4th Ed. vol I. USA: McGraw-Hill, Inc, 1993: 804-21.

Actinic Cheilosis

23. Johnson TM, Sebastien TS, Lowe L, Nelson BR. Carbon dioxide laser treatment of actinic cheilitis. Clinicohistopathologic correlation to determine the optimal depth of destruction. J Am Acad Dermatol 1992; 27:737-40.
24. Picascia DD, Robinson J. Actinic cheilitis: a review of the etiology, differential diagnosis and treatment. J Am Acad Dermatol 1987; 17:255-64.
25. Zelicson BD, Roenigk RK. Actinic cheilitis : treatment with de carbon dioxide laser. Cancer 1990; 65:1307-11.

Oral Lichen Planus

26. Allen C. Is lichen planus really premalignant? Oral Surg Oral Med Oral Pathol 1998; 85:347.
27. Andreasen JO. Oral lichen planus. I. A clinical evaluation of 115 cases. Oral Surg Oral Med Oral Pathol 1968; 25:31-42.
28. Barnard N, Scully C, Evenson J, Cunningham S, Porter S. Oral cáncer development in patients with oral lichen planus. J Oral Pathol Med 1993; 22 : 421-24.
29. Brown R, Bottomley W, Puente F, Lavigne G. A retrospective evaluation of 193 patients with oral lichen planus. J Oral Pathol Med 1993; 22: 69-72.
30. Cerero R, Llanes F, Esparza G, Bascones A, Seoane J. Displasia en liquen plano oral. Comunicación en I Congreso Europeo de Medicina Oral. Madrid. Octubre 1991.
31. Cribier B, Frances C, Chosidow O. Treatment of Lichen Planus. An Evidence-based Medicine Analysis of Efficacy. Arch Dermatol 1998; 134:1521-30.
32. De Jong WF, Albrecht M, Bánoczy J, Van der Waal I. Epithelial dysplasia in oral lichen planus. A preliminar report of a Dutch-Hungarian study of 100 cases. J Oral Surg 1984; 13:221-5.
33. Jontell M,Watts S ,Wallström M, Levin l, Sloberg K. Human papilloma virus in erosive oral lichen planus. J Oral Pathol Med 1990; 19:273-7.
34. Kaplan B, Barnes L. Oral lichen planus and squamous cell carcinoma (Case report and update of the literature). Arch Otolaryngol 1985; 111:547-7.
35. Krutchkoff DJ, Cutler L, Laskowsky S. Oral lichen planus: the evidence regarding potential malignat transformation. J Oral Pathol 1878; 7:1-7.
36. Krutchoff DJ, Eisemberg E. Lichenoid dysplasia. A distinct histopathologic entity. Oral Surg Oral Med Oral Pathol 1985; 60: 308-15.
37. Lind P, Stromme Koppang H, Aas E. Malignant transformation in oral lichen planus. Int J Oral Surg 1985; 14:509-16.
38. Lovas J, Harsany B, Elgeneidy A. Oral lichenoid dysplasia: a clinicopathologic analysis. Oral Surg Oral Med Oral Pathol 1989; 68:57-63.
39. Marder MZ, Deesen KC. Transformation of oral lichen planus to squamous cell carcinoma: a literature review and report of case. J Am Dent Assoc 1982; 105:55-60.
40. Odykoya O, Gallagher G, Shklar G. A histologic study of epithelial dysplasia in oral lichen planus. Arch Dermatol 1985; 121:1132-6.

41. Pogrel MA, Weldom LL. Carcinoma arising in erosive lichen planus in the midline of the dorsum of the tongue. Oral Surg 1983; 55:62-6.
42. Reisman RJ, Schwartz AE, Friedman EW, Gerry RG. The malignant potential of oral lichen planus-diagnostic pitfalls. Oral Surg Oral Med Oral Pathol 1974; 38:227-32.
43. Scully C, El-Kom M. Lichen Planus: review and update on pathogenesis. J Oral Pathol 1985, 14:431-58.
44. Seoane J, Vazquez J, Romero MA, Aguado A, Pomareda M. Fotoquimioterapia en el tratamiento del liquen erosivo oral. Acta Otorrinolaring 1997; 48:251-53.
45. Thorn JJ, Holmstrup P, Rindum J, Pindborg JJ. Course of various clinical forms of oral lichen planus. A propective follow-up study of 611 patients. J Oral Pathol 1988; 17:213-18.
46. Zhang L, Michelsen C, Cheng X, Zeng T, Priddy R, Rosin MP. Molecular analysis of oral lichen planus. A premalignant lesion? Am J Pathol 1997; 151:323-7.

Lupus Erythematosus

47. Bermejo A. Etiopatogenia, patología clínica con especial referencia a la mucosa bucal. Av Odontoestomatol 1991; 7:525-37.
48. Callen JP. Mucocutaneous changes in patients with lupus erythematosus : The relationship of these lesions to systemic disease. Rheum Dis Clin North Am 1988; 14:79-97.

Immunosuppression

49. Biggar RJ, Burnett W, Mikl J, Nasca P. Cancer among New York men at risk of acquired immunodeficiency syndrome. Int J Cancer 1989; 43: 979-85.
50. Blohme I, Larko O. Premalignant and malignant skin lesions in renal transplant patients. Transplantation 1984; 37 (2):165-67.
51. Diz Dios P, Oñate Sánchez R, Castro Ferreiro M, et al. Oral neoplasms in AIDS: A clinical approach for general dental practitioners. Stoma 1995; 34:7-13.
52. Epstein JB, Scully C. Neoplastic disease in the head and neck of patients with AIDS. Int J Oral Maxillofac Surg 1992; 21:219-26.
53. Flaitz CM, Nichols CM, Adler-Storthz K, Hicks MJ. Intraoral squamous cell carcinoma in human immunodeficiency virus infection. Oral Surg Oral Med Oral Pathol Oral Radiol Endod 1995; 80: 55-62.
54. Peris Z, Tiz A. Precancerous conditions and carcinomas in patients on immunosuppressive therapy. Chir Maxillofac Plast 1988; 18 (1-3): 29-32.
55. Taylor AE, Shuster S. Skin cancer after renal transplantation: the causal role of azathioprine. Acta Derm Venereol 1992; 72 (2): 115-19.

Oral Submucous Fibrosis

56. Borle RM, Borle SR. Management of oral submucous fibrosis: a conservative approach. J Oral Maxillofac Surg 1991; 49(8): 788-91.
57. Jian XC. Clinical investigation of oral submucous fibrosis. Chung Hua Kou Chiang Hsueh Tsa Chin 1989; 24(5): 299-302.
58. Maher R, Lee AJ, Warnakulasuriya KA, Lewis JA, Johnson NW. Role of areca nut in the causation of oral submucous fibrosis: a case-control study in Pakistan. J Oral Path Med 1994; 23(2): 65-69.
59. Murti PR, Bhonsole RB, Gupta PC, Daftary DK, Pindborg JJ, Mehta FS. Etiology of oral submucous fibrosis with special reference to the role of areca nut chewing. J Oral Path Med 1995; 24(4): 145-52.
60. Murti PR, Bhonsole RB, Pindborg JJ, Daftary DK, Gupta PC, Mehta FS. Malignant transformation rate in oral submucous fibrosis over a 17-year period. Community Dent Oral Epidemiol 1985; 13 (6): 340-41.
61. Pillai R, Balaram P, Reddiar KS. Pathogenisis of oral submucous fibrosis. Relationship to risk factors associated with oral cancer. Cancer 1992; 69(8): 2011-20.
62. Pindborg JJ, Murti PR, Bhonsole RB, Gupta PC, Daftary DK, Mehta FS. Oral submucous fibrosis as a precancerous condition. Scand J Dent Res 1984; 92(3): 224-29.

63. Rajendran, R. Oral submucous fibrosis: etiology, pathogenesis, and future research. Bull WHO 1994; 72 (6): 985-96.

Xeroderma Pigmentosum

64. Jain VK, Dashore A, Dixit VB. Xeroderma pigmentosum - report of four cases. Ann Dent 1989; 48 (1): 25-27.
65. Kraemer KH, Lee MM, Scotto J. Early onset of skin and oral cavity neoplasms in xeroderma pigmentosum. Lancet 1982; 1 (8262): 56-57.
66. Patton LL, Valdez IH. Xeroderma pigmentosum: review and report of a case. Oral Surg Oral Med Oral Pathol 1991; 71 (3): 297-300.

Sideropenic Dysphagia

67. Adlington P, Leedham P, Smith P. The place of iron deficiency in the Paterson-Brown-Kelly syndrome. J Laringol Otol 1973; 87 (9): 845-59.
68. Chen TS, Chen PS. Rise and fall of the Plummer-Vinson syndrome. J Gastroenterol Hepatol 1994; 9 (6): 654-58.
69. Hoeksema P E. Kelly-Paterson syndrome end carcinoma. ORL 1973; 35 (3-4): 167-70.
70. Kharrat F, Mnif S, Kechaou MS et al. La dysphagie sideropenique. Journal de Radiologie 1989; 70 (10): 563-67.
71. Khosla SN. Cricoid webs - incidence and follow-up study in Indian patients. Postgrad Med J 1984; 60 (703): 346-48.
72. Larsson LG, Sandstrom A, Westling P. Relationship of Plummer-Vinson disease to cancer of the upper alimentary tract in Sweden. Cancer Res 1975; 35: 3308-16.
73. Ramanjaneyulu P. Postcricoid cancer. Journal Medical Libanais 1974; 27 (3): 299-304.
74. Suzaki K. A roentgenological study on Plummer-Vinson syndrome. Its nature and effect of iron therapy. Journal of the Japan Broncho-esophagological Society 1983; 34 (3): 20-30.
75. Suzaki K. Carcinoma of the hypopharynx and cervical esophagus associated with Plummer-Vinson syndrome, with special reference to precancerous condition. Rinsho Hoshasen 1983; 28 (12): 1453-59.

Oral Precancer Related to Reverse Smoking

76. Mehta FS, Bhonsole RB, Murti PR, Daftary DK, Gupta PC, Pindborg JJ. Central papillary atrophy of the tongue among bidi smokers in India: a 10-year study of 182 lesions. J Oral Pathol Med 1989; 18 (8): 475-80.
77. Mehta FS, Jalsanavalla PN, Daftary DK, Gupta PC, Pindborg JJ. Reverse smoking in Andhra Pradesh, India: variability of clinical and histologic appearances of palatal changes. Int J Oral Surg 1977; 6 (2): 75-83.
78. Mercado-Ortiz G, Wilson D, Jiang DJ. Reverse smoking and palatal mucosal changes in Filipino women. Epidemiological features. Aus Dent J 1996; 41 (5): 300-303.
79. Van der Eb MM, Leyten EM, Gavarasana S, Vandenbroucke JP, Kahn PM, Cleton FJ. Reverse smoking as a risk for palatal cancer: a cross-sectional study in rural Andhra Pradesh, India. Int J Cancer 1993; 54 (5): 754-58.

Syphilis

80. Dickenson AJ, Currie WJ, Avery BS. Screening for syphilis in patients with carcinoma of the tongue. Br J oral Maxillofac Surg 1995; 33 (5):319-20.
81. Ficarra G, Zaragoza AM, Stendari L, Parri F, Cockerell CJ. Early oral presentation of lues maligna in a patient with HIV infection. A case report. Oral Surg Oral Med Oral Pathol 1993; 75 (6):728-32.
82. Michalek Am, Mahoney MC, McLaughlin CC, Murphy D, Metzger BB. Historical and contemporary correlates of syphilis and cancer. Int J Epidemiol 1994; 23 (2):381-85.
83. Ramírez-Amador V, Madero JG, Pedraza LE et al. Oral secondary syphilis in a patient with human immunodeficiency virus infection. Oral Surg Oral Med Oral Pathol Oral Radiol Endod 1996; 81 (6):652-54.
84. Schofer H, Imhof M, Thoma-Greber E et al. Active syphilis in HIV infection: a multicentre retrospective survey. The German AIDS Study Group (GASD). Genitourin Med 1996; 72 (3):176-81.

CHAPTER 7

Surgical Management of Oral Tongue Carcinoma

Po Wing Yuen, William Ignace Wei

INTRODUCTION

Carcinoma of tongue is a common head and neck cancer. High incidence can be found in areas of high consumption of tobacco, alcohol and betal squid. In Hong Kong, tongue cancer accounts for 0.7% of all new cases of cancer, and the age standardised incidence per 100,000 population is 2.6 for males and 1.3 for females.[1] The incidence of oral cancer in Hong Kong is, however, ten times less common than in India which is 24.2 per 100,000 population for males and 11.2 per 100,000 population for females.[2]

The development of cancer is now believed to be a multi-step process with accumulation of many genetic abnormalities. The common genetic abnormalities in tongue carcinoma includes mutation and overexpression of oncogenes, tumour suppressor genes and other apoptosis related genes.[3-4] As a result of these genetic abnormalities, the tongue epithelial cells proliferate out of control. The progressive development of cancer sometimes appears clinically in its premalignant stage as leukoplakia or erythroplakia.[5] These intermediate steps of cancer formation appear histologically as dysplasia. With further accumulation of genetic abnormalities involved in cancer development, the epithelial cells become cancer cells which can invade and metastasise. Carcinoma of tongue appears as non-healing painful ulceration mostly at the lateral border of tongue. (Fig. 7.1, Plate 6) shows a patient with ulcerative carcinoma with surrounding leuko-plakia.

TNM Stage of Oral Tongue Carcinoma, AJCC/UICC 1997

Primary Tumour (T)

Tx	primary tumour cannot be assessed
T0	no evidence of primary tumour
Tis	carcinoma *in situ*
T1	tumour $\leq$ 2 cm in greatest dimension
T2	tumour > 2 cm but $\leq$ 4 cm in greatest dimension
T3	tumour > 4 cm in greatest dimension

T4 tumour invades adjacent structures (e.g., through cortical bone, into deep extrinsic muscle of tongue, maxillary sinus, skin; superficial erosion of bone/tooth socket by gingival primary is not sufficient to classify as T4)

Regional Lymph Nodes (N)

Nx	regional lymph nodes cannot be assessed
N0	no regional lymph node metastasis
N1	metastasis in single ipsilateral node, ≤ 3 cm in greatest dimension
N2a	metastasis in single ipsilateral node, > 3 cm but ≤ 6 cm
N2b	metastasis in multiple ipsilateral nodes, all ≤ 6 cm
N2c	metastasis in bilateral or contralateral nodes, all ≤ 6 cm
N3	metastasis in lymph node > 6 cm in greatest dimension

Distant Metastasis (M)

Mx	distant metastasis cannot be assessed
M0	no distant metastasis
M1	distant metastasis

Stage

0	Tis N0 M0
I	T1 N0 M0
II	T2 N0 M0
III	T3 N0 M0, T1-2 N1 M0, T3 N1 M0
IV	T4 N0-1 M0, any T N2-3 M0, any T any N M1

TREATMENT OPTIONS

The treatment of oral tongue carcinoma remains controversial. Radiotherapy and surgery are each used as primary treatment by radiation oncologists and surgeons.[6-13] The results of radiotherapy and surgery are similar for early stage carcinoma. It is, however, more common practice to treat stage I and II carcinomas with surgery alone and stage III and IV carcinomas with combined surgery and radiotherapy.

Sites of Treatment Failures

In order to improve treatment results, we have to understand the causes and sites of treatment failures. In a retrospective study of 112 patients who had primary surgical treatment of oral tongue carcinomas in the Department of Surgery, the University of Hong Kong, the first sites of tumour recurrence were 10 (9%) local, 25 (22%) nodal, 3 (3%) locoregional, 5 (5%) distant, 1 (1%) local and distant, 3 (3%) nodal and distant, and one (1%) neck extranodal site.[12] The median time of first appearance of recurrence after operation was 7 months (range 6 weeks to 58 months, mean 10 months, 90% within 22 months).

Over 90% treatment failures were due to local or regional lymph node recurrences. Further improvement of treatment result, therefore, mainly depends on whether we can have better local and nodal control of the cancer.

Local Control

Local recurrence accounts for about 15% of treatment failures. The median time to local recurrence after operation was 8 months (range 2-58 months, mean 12 months). The 5-year actuarial local control rates were T1 79%, T2 81%, T3 91% and T4 60%. There were no significant differences in the actuarial local control rates for T1 to T3, but the actuarial local control rate was significantly lower in T4 patients compared with T1 to T3.[13]

It has been shown that there is high risk of local recurrence despite adjuvant radiotherapy for patients with positive resection margin.[14-15] There is also very little chance of successful salvage of local recurrence by surgery.[16-17] In a literature review of local recurrence after glossectomy, of all 104 patients with local recurrence after glossectomy, only 18% patients can be successfully salvaged.[17] It is, therefore, important to ensure adequate initial surgical resection of the tumour rather than relying on adjuvant radiotherapy or subsequent surgical salvage for the residual tumour left behind.

Histological examination of resection margins by frozen section at operation is always recommended. Unfortunately, frozen section often does not detect the subclinical local residual tumour. Accurate tumour size assessment together with adequate resection remains essential for the surgical management of these patients.

Surgical Margin

The surgical techniques of tumour resection vary from partial glossectomy, hemiglossectomy to subtotal and total glossectomy. Additional resection of larynx, tonsils and mandible are necessary in more advanced cancer. Irrespective to the techniques of surgery, the aim of surgical resection is to achieve reasonably clear resection. Tumour is a three-dimensional structure, and carcinoma of tongue spreads in three-dimensional planes. The mode and distance of local spread affect the surgical judgement on resection margin taken from the tumour edge. An optimal resection should not compromise the local control for inadequate resection or causing unnecessary functional morbidity for too much resection. The knowledge of how tumour spreads locally in the three-dimensional plane is important in the planning of surgical resection.

We have reported the modes and distance of local spread in 50 glossectomy specimens.[16] The results are summarised in Table 7.1. (Fig. 7.2, Plate 6) is an example to illustrate the presence of tumour microsatellites away from the main tumour. The distribution of the maximum distance of spread away from the tumour edge is shown in Figure 7.3. The maximum distance of local spread from the border of the main tumour was found to be 1.8 cm (mean 0.3 cm, 96% within 1.2 cm). There were no significant correlation between distance of local spread to tumour diameter, depth, and volume. The distance of spread was also not related to the pathological T-stage, and histological differentiation.[16]

Table 7.1: Mode and distance of local spread

Mode of local spread	*Incidence*	*Maximum distance of spread (cm)*
Submucosal direct spread	5 (10%)	0.6 cm
Muscular direct spread	19 (38%)	1.5 cm
Perineural	6 (12%)	0.5 cm
Submucosal microsatellite	8 (16%)	1.2 cm
Muscular microsatellite	11 (22%)	1.8 cm

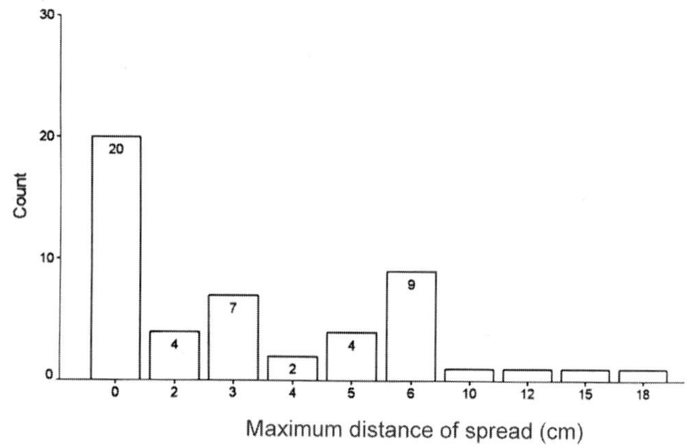

Fig. 7.3: Distance of local spread of carcinoma away from the main tumour mass

Since 95% tumour had local spread within 1.2 cm from the tumour, a clear histological resection margin could be achieved with over 95% confidence level for a 1.5 to 2 cm surgical resection margin from the tumour border. A surgical resection margin of less than 1.5 cm is not recommended as it will increase the chance for positive histological resection margin and compromises the prognosis of local control. On the other hand, more radical resection of more than 2 cm surgical resection margin can further increase the confidence of histological clear resection margin, the benefit of the radical resection, however, should be judged against the magnitude of surgical morbidity. Therefore, a 1.5 to 2 cm surgical resection margin should be an optimal choice in the treatment of oral tongue carcinoma.

Tumour Size Assessment

Although a 1.5 to 2 cm resection margin is recommended, an accurate assessment of tumour size is important. Under-estimation of tumour size will increase the chance of positive resection margin despite of an optimal 1.5 to 2 cm resection margin. Over-estimation of tumour size will result in unnecessary removal of normal tissue and jeopardises lingual function.

Clinical assessment of tumour size by palpation is not always reliable. When the clinical and pathological stages were compared, the clinical estimation of tumour stagings were correct only in 76% patients. The sizes of tumours were underestimated in 20% patients, and were overestimated in 4% patients.[18]

Radiological assessment of tumour size by using ultrasound, CT scan and MRI have been reported in the literature. In our experience, MRI is the most accurate scanning method to assess the tumour size. MRI also has advantage of taking images at three-dimensional planes which helps in the planning of resection. Figure 7.4 to 7.6 show clear images of tongue carcinoma in coronal, sagittal and axial planes.

Resection Technique

Transoral resection is adequate for small tumours. In large tumour that requires reconstruction, neck dissection should be completed before glossectomy and the tongue can be delivered to the

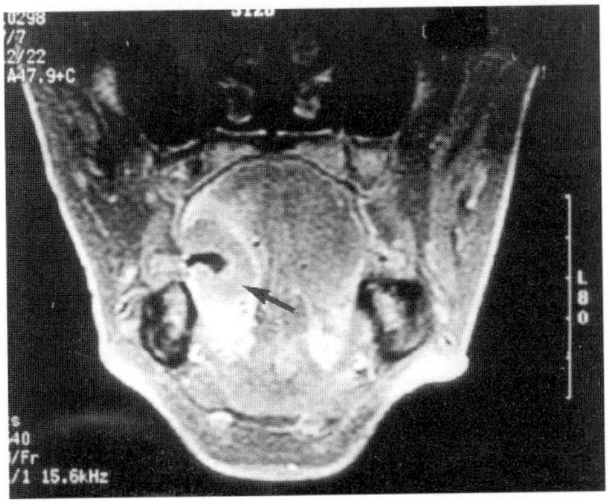

Fig. 7.4: MRI coronal scan of ulcerative carcinoma over right lateral border of tongue (arrow)

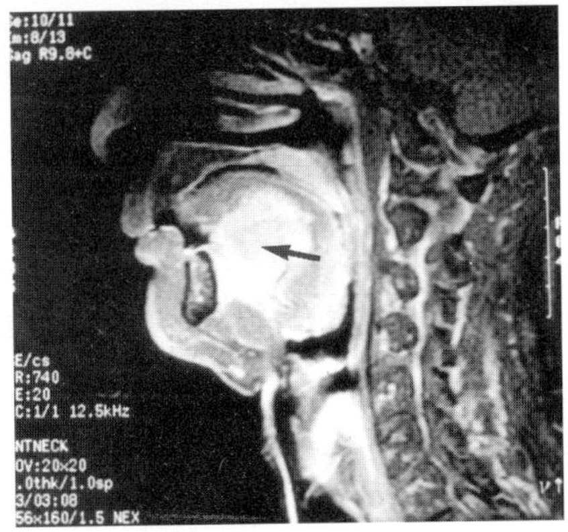

Fig. 7.5: MRI sagittal scan of ulcerative carcinoma over right lateral border of tongue (arrow)

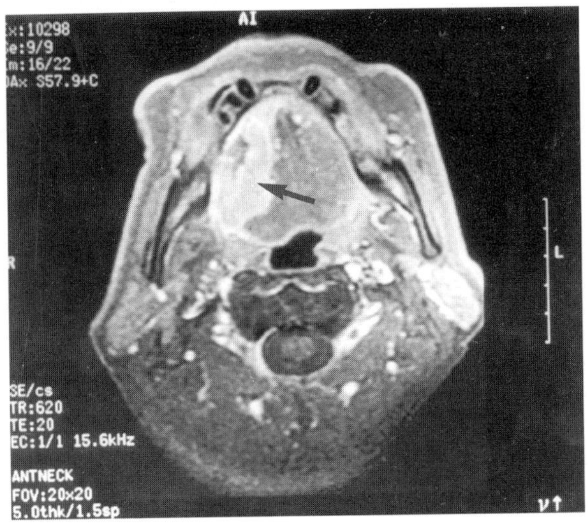

Fig. 7.6: MRI axial scan of ulcerative tumour over right lateral border of tongue (arrow)

neck for further resection. Before surgical resection of the tumour, the tumour should be carefully outlined with colour dye. A 1.5 to 2 cm resection margin is outlined with colour dye. It is good practice to use a ruler to measure the resection margin to make sure that you have the correct plan of resection. (Fig. 7.7, Plate 6) shows the outline of tumour and line of incision. The line of resection should then be outlined again with diathermy because the colour dye will disappear soon after you have begun dissection. The dissection is done by using a monopolar diathermy pen with careful haemostasis at each step. The tumour border should be palpated repeatedly during dissection with particular attention to the deep margin to make sure that the correct resection margin is achieved.

In patients with tongue base involvement, the larynx can often be preserved without compromising clear resection. Removal of larynx is, however, recommended even when the larynx is not involved by tumour particularly in elderly patients who cannot tolerate minimal aspiration after total glossectomy. Marginal or segmental mandibulectomy may sometimes be necessary in oral tongue cancer with presence of mandibular invasion.

Reconstruction Technique

The reconstruction method depends on the extent of resection. Primary closure is adequate for glossectomy of up to half of the tongue without significant impairment of lingual function. (Fig. 7.8, Plate 6) shows the result of primary closure. When more than half of the tongue is removed, primary closure will compromise the lingual function and flap reconstruction is necessary.

Free radial forearm skin flap is recommended for reconstruction of partial glossectomy defect in which a muscle bulk is not required. The free radial forearm flap has reliable skin vascularity and it is a thin pliable flap that can be easily fitted into the oral cavity. (Figs 7.9 and 7.10, Plate 6) show the use of free forearm flap for the reconstruction of oral defect. The radial artery and its venae comitante are anastomosed to the facial artery and vein in the submandibular region. The donor site defect can be closed primarily or can be covered with split thickness skin graft.

When free flap reconstruction technique is not available, or radical neck dissection has to be done because of nodal involvement, or total glossectomy has been done, or larynx has been removed, a pedicle pectoralis major myocutaneous flap (PM Flap) can be used. (Figs 7.11 to 7.13, Plate 7) show the reconstruction of subtotal glossectomy with PM flap. PM flap has very reliable muscle bulk which can be very useful in the reconstruction of large oral defect which a muscle bulk is required to support the floor of oral cavity. Although the skin island is less reliable with high risk of partial skin flap dehiscence or necrosis, the reliable muscle bulk can sustain leakage. Wound healing is almost always successful with conservative expectant treatment even in the presence of large superficial skin island necrosis. When a segment of mandible is removed, it can be reconstructed with pectoralis major myocutaneous flap with the underlying rib or a metal plate. Free osteocutaneous fibula flap can also be used to reconstruct the oral mucosal and bony defect when muscle bulk is not required.

Subclinical Nodal Metastasis

Tongue carcinoma has high propensity of nodal metastasis even in its early stage.[19-21] The pathological incidence of subclinical nodal metastasis for T1 and T2 oral tongue carcinoma was found to be 36% in a study by whole organ serial sectioning of 50 elective neck dissection specimens of clinically N0 neck.[18] The most common site of nodal metastasis was ipsilateral level II, and 95% metastatic nodes were found in the ipsilateral levels I, II, III. Contralateral nodal metastasis and contralateral nodal recurrence were found only in less than 5% patients.[21]

In our study, 36% patients were found to have radiologically undetectable micrometastasis in the neck.[21] Most subclinical positive nodes only contained tiny focal micrometastasis within the lymph nodes or on the capsular lymphatic vessels. The median size of the micrometastasis was only 3 mm in diameter and these cancer cells occupied a median of only 6% of nodal cross-sectional areas. An example of subclinical micrometastasis is shown in the capsular lymphatic of a 1 cm neck node in (Fig. 7.14, Plate 7). There were numerous subclinical normal lymph nodes in the neck, the median total number of lymph nodes were 48 in the surgical

Plate 6

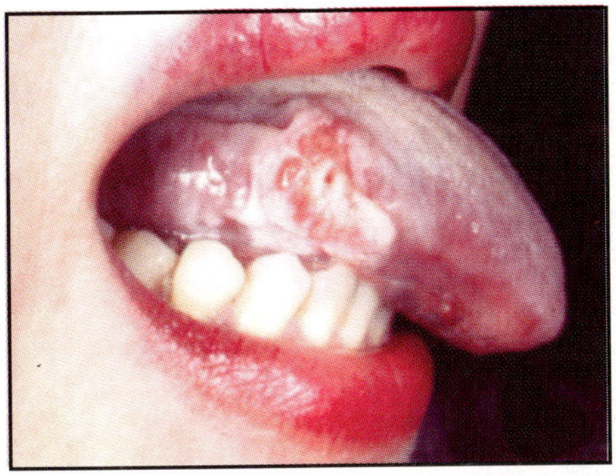

Fig. 7.1: Ulcerative carcinoma over the lateral border of tongue with surrounding leukoplakia

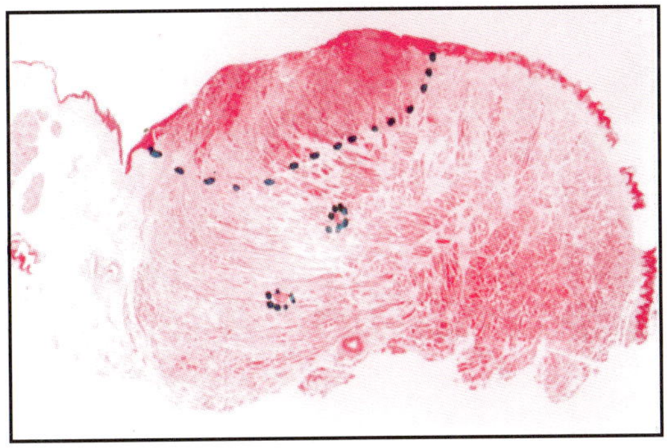

Fig. 7.2: Local spread of carcinoma, 2 clusters of carcinoma cells can be seen away from the main tumour mass (outlined with dots)

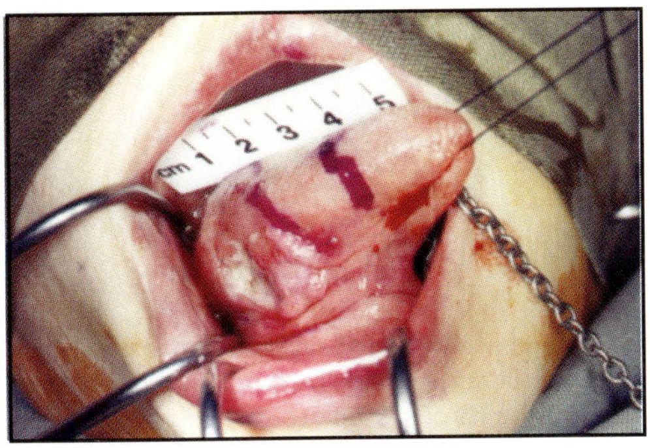

Fig. 7.7: Outlining of tumour border and resection line with colour dye

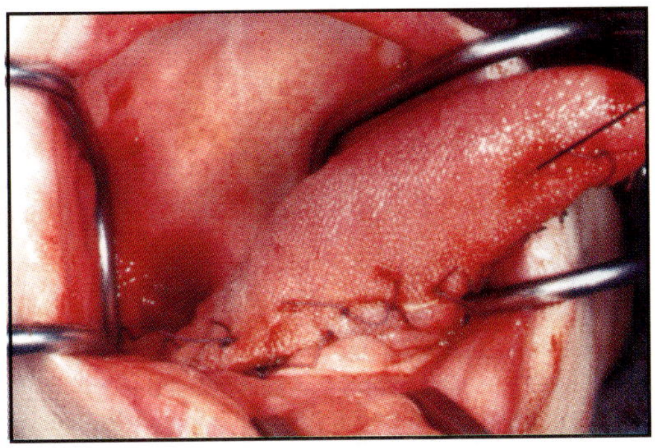

Fig. 7.8: Primary closure after partial glossectomy

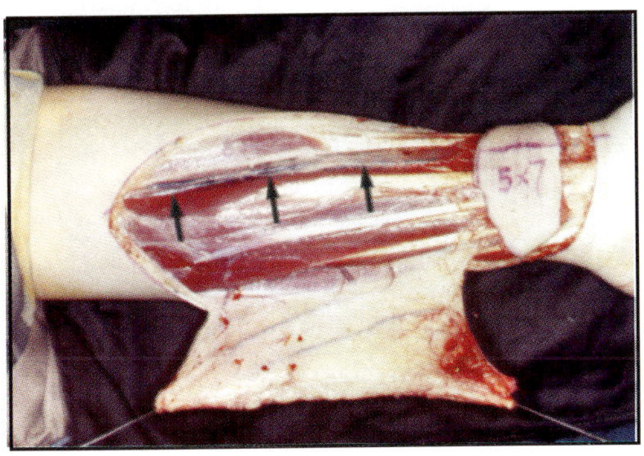

Fig. 7.9: Free radial forearm flap is harvested from the distal end of forearm, the radial artery and its vein commitents are used for the vascular anastomosis (arrows)

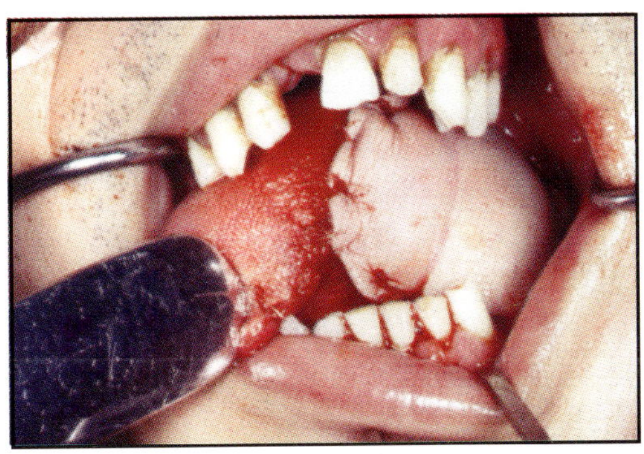

Fig. 7.10: Free radial forearm flap is used in the reconstruction of left glossectomy defect in the oral cavity

Plate 7

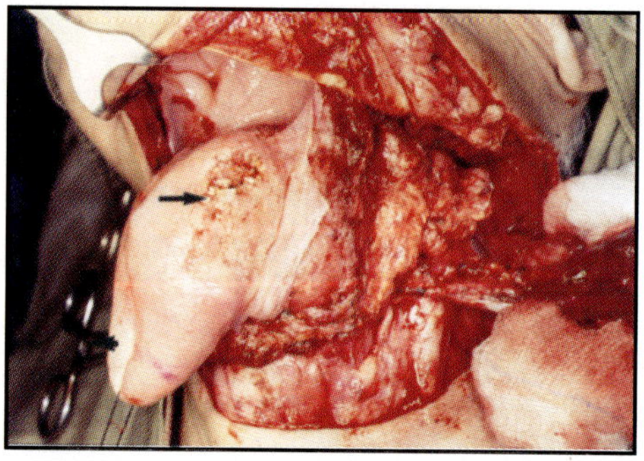

Fig. 7.11: A large tumour over left lateral border of tongue requires subtotal glossectomy, the whole tongue is delivered to the neck for further resection (arrow)

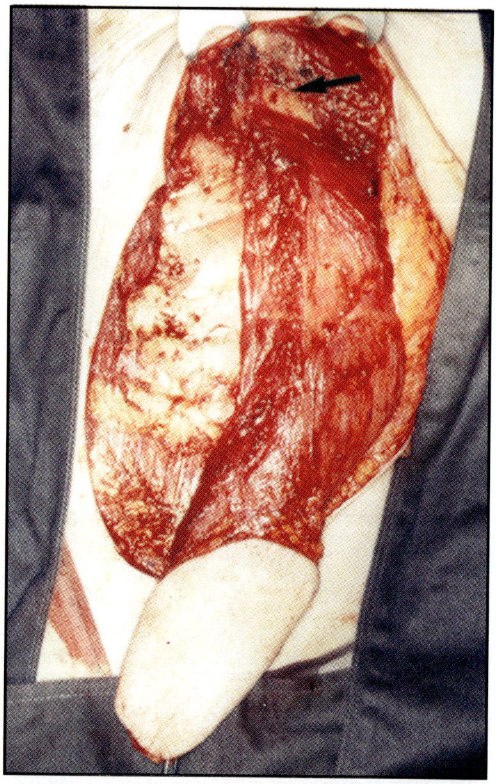

Fig. 7.12: A left PM flap is harvested, it is an island flap with the clavicular part of the pectoralis muscle being divided to expose the vascular pedicle (arrow)

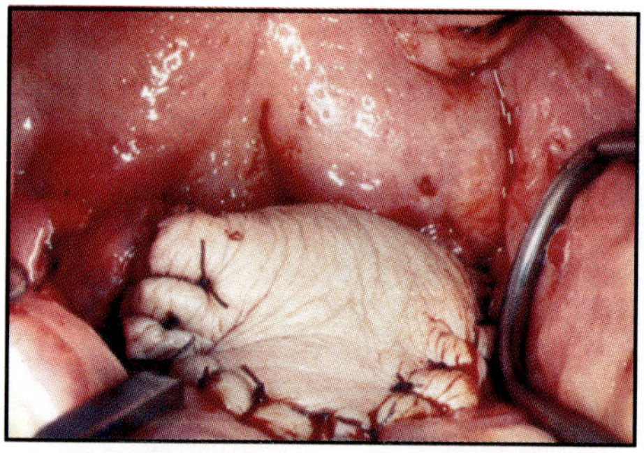

Fig. 7.13: The island PM flap is used in the reconstruction of the floor of mouth after subtotal glossectomy

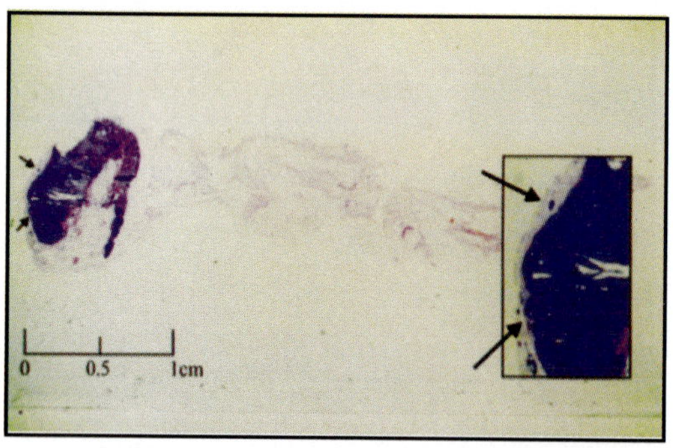

Fig. 7.14: Micrometastasis in the capsular lymphatics of a 1 cm subclinical neck node (arrows)

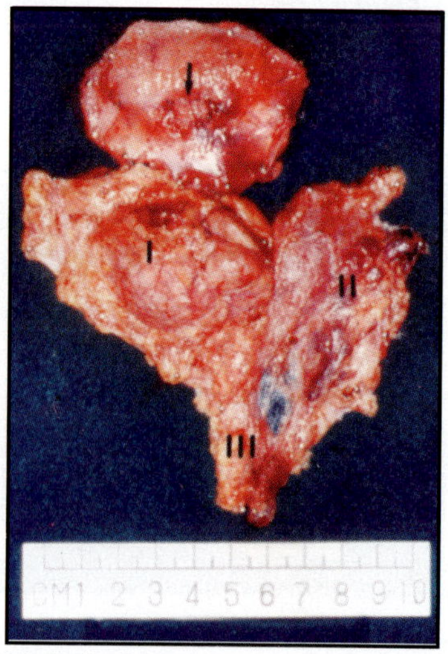

Fig. 7.15: Left glossectomy and left selective I,II,III neck dissection specimen, ulcerative tumour (arrow) is seen at the left lateral border of tongue

specimens and was up to 140. Since only 1% nodes contained micrometastasis, the small percentage of metastatic nodes together with the small size of the micrometastasis amidst the large number of normal nodes in the neck would cause tremendous difficulty in the detection of subclinical nodal metastasis pre-operatively.[21]

Although pre-operative radiological screening including CT scan, MRI or ultrasound-guided aspiration cytology became our routine work-up protocol nowadays, these radiological screening methods are useful but not adequate in detecting those micrometastasis inside the small non-palpable nodes.[21] All available pre-operative imaging modalities including CT scan, MRI, and ultrasound-guided fine needle aspiration cytology cannot replace the role of elective neck dissection as an accurate diagnostic procedure for staging of the N0 neck. The incidence of nodal recurrence will remain high if the radiologically N0 necks are not treated electively.

Although intra-operative sampling with frozen section may help occasionally in the detection of micrometastasis, the same difficulties due to the large number of normal nodes and the small size of micrometastasis persisted as in pre-operative imaging. The intra-operative sampling with frozen section is sometimes useful but not adequate in the detection of micrometastasis.[21] The only indication for the intra-operative sampling is when the surgeon is prepared to proceed to radical neck dissection upon finding a positive node. Since we will not proceed to radical neck dissection upon finding metastatic node intra-operatively, we have lost the interest in taking intra-operative frozen section of lymph nodes recently. We rely more on post-operative radiotherapy to eradicate the possible residual micrometastasis in the neck. Intra-operative frozen section of nodes is, however, still recommended in conditions when post-operative radiotherapy will not be given such as in patients with prior radiotherapy to the neck; in such situation, the finding of positive node by intra-operative frozen section can help us to go ahead for radical neck dissection.

Elective Neck Dissection for N0 Neck

The treatment of N0 neck of early stage I and stage II oral tongue carcinoma is controversial, both elective neck dissection and 'watchful waiting policy' have their proponents in different centres.[22-30]

We have shown in a retrospective study that elective neck dissection has significant benefit in the improvement of regional control and long-term survival.[22] Of the 63 N0 neck patients being studied, the regional recurrence rates were 47% for 'watchful waiting', 9% for elective neck dissection (0% for elective radical neck dissection, 13% for elective selective I, II, III neck dissection). The reduction of regional recurrences was statistically significant for elective neck dissection. Both elective radical neck dissection and elective selective I, II, III neck dissection had better regional control compared with the 'watchful waiting'. The 13% difference in regional recurrence rate between elective radical neck dissection and elective selective I, II, III neck dissection is not statistically significant.

In our study, no patient died of regional recurrence after elective radical neck dissection. The regional recurrence-related mortality rates were 23% for 'watchful waiting', 3% for elective neck dissection (0% for elective radical neck dissection, 4% for elective selective I, II, III neck dissection). The 20% difference in regional recurrence related mortality rates between 'watchful waiting' and elective neck dissection was statistically significant. The 23% difference of regional recurrence-related mortality rate between 'watchful waiting' and elective radical neck dissection was statistically not significant probably due to the small sample size. The 19% difference of regional recurrence-related mortality rate between 'watchful waiting' and elective selective I, II, III neck dissection was statistically not significant probably also due to the small sample size. The 4% difference in regional recurrence-related mortality between elective radical neck dissection and elective selective neck dissection was not significant.

From the results of this study, we can conclude that elective neck dissection can reduce both initial regional recurrence rate and eventual regional recurrence-related mortality, and it also has long-term survival benefit. There is no significant difference in the treatment results between elective radical neck dissection and elective selective I, II, III neck dissection. Elective ipsilateral selective I, II, III neck dissection is, therefore, a treatment strategy of choice for clinically N0 neck of oral tongue carcinoma.

Selective neck dissection of the ipsilateral I, II, III nodes can be done after glossectomy. In most early carcinoma in which the glossectomy defect can be closed primarily, it is not necessary to perform glossectomy and neck dissection en-bloc. After primary closure of the glossectomy defect, a horizontal neck incision can be used to approach the level I, II, III nodes. (Fig. 7.15, Plate 7) shows the glossectomy and ipsilateral level I, II, III neck specimens.

CONCLUSIONS

The management of tongue carcinoma can be improved with better understanding of the behaviour of the cancer and problems of our treatment strategy. Local control can be improved with pre-operative assessment of tumour size by using MRI and careful planing of resection with a 1.5 to 2 cm resection margin. Nodal control can be improved by elective ipsilateral selective I, II, III neck dissection. With better locoregional control of tongue cancer, the long-term survival will be improved.

REFERENCES

1. Hong Kong Cancer Registry Annual Statistical Report. Hospital Authority 1989; p.27-28.
2. Sankaranarayanan R, Nair K, Mathew B, et al. Recent results of oral cancer research in Kerala, India. Head Neck 1992; 14:107-12.
3. Ogden GR, Kiddie RA, Lunny DP, Lane DP. Assessment of p53 protein expression in normal. Benign, and malignant oral mucosa. J Path 1992; 166:389-94.
4. Schoelch ML, Le QT, Silverman S, McMillan A, Dekker NP, Fu KK, Ziober BL, Regezi JA. Apoptosis associated proteins and the development of oral squamous cell carcinoma. Oral Oncology 1999; 35:77-85.
5. Suarez P, Batsakis JG, El-Naggar AK. Leukoplakia: still a gallimaufry or is progress being made? – a review. Advances in Anatomic Pathol 1999; 5(3):137-55.
6. Mendenhall MW, Parsons JT, Stringer SP, et al. T2 oral tongue carcinoma treated with radiotherapy: analysis of local control and complications. Radiother Oncol 1989; 16:275-81.
7. Padmanabhan TK, Sankaranarayanan R, Nair MK. Evaluation of local control, survival and pattern of failure with radiotherapy in cancer of the tongue. Oncol 1990; 47:121-23.
8. Piedbois P, Mazeron JJ, Haddad E, et al. Stage I-II squamous cell carcinoma of the oral cavity treated by iridium -192: is elective neck dissection indicated? Radiother Oncol 1991; 21:100-106.
9. Bier-Laning C, Adams GL. Patterns of recurrence after carbon dioxide laser excision of intraoral squamous cell carcinoma. Arch Otolaryngol Head Neck Surg. 1995; 121:1239-44.
10. Franceschi D, Gupta R, Spiro RH, Shah JP. Improved survival in the treatment of squamous carcinoma of the oral tongue. Am J Surg 1993; 166:360-65.
11. Lydiatt DD, Robbins KT, Byers RM, Wolf PF. Treatment of stage I and II oral tongue cancer. Head Neck 1993; 15:308-12.

12. Yuen APW, Wei WI, Wong YM, Tang KC. Comprehensive analysis of results of surgical treatment of oral tongue carcinoma in Hong Kong. Chinese Med J 1997; 110(11): 859-64.
13. Yuen APW, Wei WI, Lam LK, Ho WK, Kwong D. Results of surgical salvage of locoregional recurrence of carcinoma of tongue after radiotherapy failure. Ann Otol Rhino Laryngol. 1997; 106:779-82.
14. Loree TR, Strong EW. Significance of positive margins in oral cavity squamous cell carcinoma. Am J Surg 1990; 260:410-14.
15. van Es RJJ, van Nieuw Amerongen N, Slootweg PJ, Egyedi P. Resection margin as a predictor of recurrence at the primary site for T1 and T2 oral cancers. Arch Otorhinolaryngol Head Neck Surg 1996; 122:521-25.
16. Yuen APW, Lam KY, Chan ACL, Wei WI, Lam LK. Clinicopathological analysis of local spread of carcinoma of tongue. Am J Surg 1998; 175:242-44.
17. Yuen APW, Wei WI, Wong SHW, Ng RWM. Local recurrence of carcinoma of tongue: patient prognosis. Ear Nose Throat J (in press).
18. Yuen PW. Carcinoma of tongue – clinicopathological analysis. Thesis of Master of Surgery, The University of Hong Kong, 1997.
19. Li XM, Wei WI, Guo XF, Yuen PW, Lam LK. Cervical lymph node metastasis patterns of squamous carcinomas in the upper aerodigestive tract. J Laryngol Otol. 1996; 110:937-41.
20. Ho CM, Lam KH, Wei WI, et al. Occult lymph node metastasis in small oral tongue cancers. Head Neck 1992; 14:359-63.
21. Yuen APW, Lam KY, Chan CLA, Wei WI, Lam LK, Ho CM. Clinicopathological analysis of elective neck dissection for N0 neck of early oral tongue carcinoma. Am J Surg 1999; 177:90-92.
22. Yuen APW, Wei WI, Wong YM, Tang KC. Elective neck dissection versus observation in the surgical treatment of early oral tongue carcinoma. Head and Neck 1997; 19:583-88.
23. Huges CJ, Gallo O, Spiro, Shah JP. Management of occult neck metastasis in oral cavity squamous carcinoma. Am J Surg 1993; 166:380-83.
24. Jesse RH, Fletcher GH. Treatment of neck in patients with squamous cell carcinoma of head and neck. Cancer 1977; 39:868-72.
25. van den Brouck C, Sancho-Garnier H, Chassagne D, et al. Elective versus therapeutic radical neck dissection in epidermoid carcinoma of oral cavity, results of a randomized clinical trial. Cancer 1980; 46:386-90.
26. Fakih AR, Rao RS, Borges AM, Patel AR. Elective versus therapeutic neck dissection in squamous cell carcinoma of tongue: a prospective randomized study. Semin Surg Oncol 1989; 158:327-30.
27. Friedman M, Mafee MF, Pacella BL, et al. Rationale for elective neck dissection in 1990. Laryngoscope 1990; 100:54-59.
28. Henick DH, Silver CE, Heller KS, et al. Supraomohyoid neck dissection as a staging procedure for squamous cell carcinomas of the oral cavity and oropharynx. Head Neck 1995; 17:119-23.
29. Silver CE, Moisa II. Elective treatment of the neck in cancer of the oral tongue. Seminars Surg Oncol 1991; 7:14-19.
30. O'Brien CJ, Lahr CJ, Soong SJ, et al. Surgical treatment of early stage carcinoma of the oral tongue-would adjuvant treatment be beneficial? Head Neck Surg 1986; 8:401-08.

CHAPTER 8

Obstructive Sleep Apnoea

Janardhan Rao J, Vinay Kumar EC, Sathavahana Chowdary V

INTRODUCTION

Obstructive sleep apnoea (OSA) was well described in the classic pickwickian syndrome in Charles Dicken's classic work "The pick wick papers".

Though this has had passing references in medical literature in the past few decades, it was only in the past 15 years or so that sleep disorders (and specifically OSA) became well recognised entities.

As physicians become more and more aware of the ill effects of severe snoring and obstructive sleep apnoea, there are more concerted efforts to find ways of dealing with this condition.

It is now universally accepted that 'Sleep Apnoea' is a potentially serious medical condition. Since 95% of apnoeas are obstructive and since obstruction is in the upper airway, we as Otolaryngologists are directly concerned with the diagnosis and management of this important sleep disorder.

DEFINITIONS

Sleep apnoea can be defined as cessation of airflow at the level of nostrils and mouth lasting at least 10 seconds. Sleep apnoea can be classified into three types:

Obstructive

No airflow, but, continued respiratory effort; obstruction being anywhere from nose to larynx.

Central

No airflow, and no respiratory efforts; the cause is believed to be at brainstem level.

Mixed

No airflow or effort for atleast 10 seconds, followed by continued absence of airflow but measureable respiratory effort. Majority of apnoeas are obstructive and pure central apnoeas are very rare.

A patient is said to be having obstructive sleep apnoea syndrome (OSAS) if he has more than five apnoeas per hour of sleep or more than 30 apnoeas in seven hours of sleep. Number of apnoeas per hour is called apnoeic index. Apnoeas can be mild (5-20 per hour), moderate (21-30 per hour) or severe (more than 30 apnoeas per hour).

CLINICAL PICTURE

Loud snoring is the most common or many a time the only symptom of obstructive sleep apnoea. According to American studies 3/4th of loud snorers have some degree of apnoea. The other symptoms are profound excessive daytime sleepiness (EDS), reduced sleep latency, morning headaches, repeated arousals from sleep and abnormal movements during sleep. The associated problems can be personality changes, sexual impotence, intellectual deterioration, hypertension and cardiopulmonary sequelae. Many of these can be explained by oxygen de-saturation during apnoeic spells. Some of the known diseases which can cause OSAS are adenotonsillar hypertrophy, nasopharyngeal angiofibroma, tumours of pharynx, vocal cord paralysis and hypothyroidism. OSAS is more common in males and predominantly a disease of obese people.

The obstructive segment in OSAS can be anywhere in the nose, pharynx and larynx. The various sites can be classified as follows:

- Level – I : Nose and nasopharynx.
- Level – II : Velopharyngeal sphincter and soft palate.
- Level – III : Base of tongue and superior hypopharynx.
- Level – IV : Larynx and inferior hypopharynx.

CLINICAL APPROACH

A careful history and clinical examination forms an important approach to the proper diagnosis of sleep apnoea syndrome.

It is important that the sleeping partner is present during the history taking and the time spent at this stage could reveal the severity of the problem. The clinical examination helps to diagnose any underlying disease like hypothyroidism, bilateral vocal cord palsy, nasal polypi, tumours, etc. and any associated diseases like hypertension and to indicate level(s) of obstruction. In paediatric population adenotonsillar hypertrophy and nasal problems are common conditions causing OSA.

In the first stance the following investigations are done:

1. General investigations.
2. Thyroid profile.
3. Cephalometry.

General investigations help us to assess the general condition of the patient and to diagnose any associated diseases like diabetes, hypercholesteraemia, pulmonary problems, etc.

Hypothyroidism is an important and common disorder which predisposes a patient to OSA. Thyroid screening must be done routinely for all patients of OSA.

Cephalometry

Cephalometric analysis gives us valuable information as to the size of the airway, the bulkiness of the surrounding soft tissues and the anatomical bony abnormalities.

X-Ray Cephalogram

Cephalograms are done using a panex—EC (cephalo), an X-ray machine devised for orthopantogram and cephalogram.

Lateral cephalograms are taken in sitting position. The subject is given mouthful of barium paste and is asked to roll it up in the oral cavity and swallow it. The purpose of barium application is for better delineation of soft tissue landmarks. The head is positioned in the head holder and a 2 mm thick cardboard is placed between the jaws. The subject is asked to occlude the jaw and to exhale gently during the exposure of the film.

The next step is to trace the landmarks on the graph paper from the cephalogram film. The cephalogram film represents the skull lateral view with almost zero magnification factor. The following landmarks were pointed and used for evaluation of various parameters.

Sub spinale: The deepest point on the premaxillary contour between anterior nasal spine and central incisors.

Gn.Gnathion: The most outward and everted point on the mandibular symphysis.

G.Genial tubercle: The most posterior point on the mandibular symphysis.

Go-Gonion: The point defining the angle of the mandibular symphysis.

PNS: Posterior nasal spine.

H.: The most anterosuperior point on the body of the hyoid bone.

TT: Tongue apex.

Cephalometric variables were used to measure the:

1. Soft palate area and distance from soft palate to posterior pharynngeal wall.
2. Tongue area in relation to oral cavity, tongue base area projecting into oropharynx and the distance between tongue base and posterior pharyngeal wall.
3. Angle of Gnathion, Gonion and Hyoid which indicates position of hyoid in relation to tongue base.

C.T Cephalometry Topogram Technique

This is the new technique we are following presently. The patient is asked to lie on the CT scan table top in a natural sleeping supine position, head is fixed in the head holder with frankfurt plane approximately perpendicular to the horizontal plane. Mouthful of barium paste is given and the patient is asked to swallow.

A topogram is planned—Topogram is a scan which is done on a running table top cranio-caudally. The patient is breathing normally during the scan. After achieving a good quality topogram, the evaluation of all the parameters are done by the same method followed on X-ray cephalogram.

The advantages of C.T Cephalogram (Topographic) are:

1. The natural sleeping supine posture of the patient as against the standing/sitting posture required on X-ray cephalogram.
2. Easy to perform the topogram.
3. Easy to measure the parameters on CT console.
4. Magnification of the particular anatomical landmark is possible to represent the pathology.
5. Good quality multiformat images.

The normal values derived after a control study in our hospital are used for evaluation. Tables 8.1 and 8.2 show the control values of various parameters.

Table 8.1

	Normal values (mean S.D.)	*Suggestive abnormal value*
UA Sq.mm	221+/- 44.859	> 300 sq.mm
UP Phw.mm	11.6+/- 3.748	< 8 mm.
UT Phw.mm	11.6+/- 4.088	< 6 mm
UD mm	10.1+/- 1.729	> 8 mm

Table 8.2

	Normal values (mean S.D.)	*Suggestive abnormal value*
OCA Sq.mm	3758.1+/-453.886	—
TCA Sq.mm	2819.4+/-444.984	> 3200 Sq.mm
TBA Sq.mm	561.6+/-197.606	> 750 sq.mm
TB Phw.mm	12.65+/-5.313	< 6 mm
Gn GoH	15.9+/-6.724	> 22

The step two of investigations includes fibre-optic examination of the upper airway, poly somnography (PSG) or modified sleep study.

Fibre-Optic Examination

Flexible fibre-optic nasopharyngolaryngoscope can be used to examine the airway at nasopharyngeal and tongue base levels. The patient is asked to perform Muller's manoeuvre. Here the patient attempts a forced inspiratory effort with a partially obstructed nasal airway while we examine the airway space at level-II and level-III. In normal people airway opens during this manoeuvre, while in patients with OSA, the airway collapses. It is also useful to assess the degree of mechanical obstruction. Reduction in OSA.

Polysomnography (PSG)

The PSG is helpful in assessing the severity of disease and also in the differential diagnosis of excessive daytime somnolance (EDS). The overnight PSG has a 16 channel polygraph including EEG, EOG, ECG, submental EMG, arterial oxygen saturation, air flow oronasal thermistors and rib cage and abdominal wall motion recorders. The PSG helps in recording the number of apnoeas and hypopnoeas, differentiates obstructive from central, records sleep patterns and detects any associated cardiac abnormalities.

The other diseases which can cause EDS are (apart from OSA) narcolepsy, circadian rhythm disorder and restless legs syndrome. Modified sleep study can be done in less severe cases to save the high cost of the PSG. In this, the sleeping patient is observed by a skilled person for number and length of apnoeas while oxygen saturation is recorded by a pulse oximeter.

Upper Airway Resistance Syndrome

Upper airway resistance syndrome (UARS) is a condition halfway between pure snorers (noisemakers only) and OSA (snorers who stop breathing during sleep). In UARS the patient does not stop breathing and, therefore his oxygen level does not drop. However, the body has to perform extra work to drive the air through the narrow passage of the throat during breathing. This extra effort causes fragmentation of sleep. The persons do not necessarily wake up completely but their sleep is disrupted and often unrefreshing.

People with UARS often wake up unrefreshed, have excessive daytime sleepiness and tiredness which can lead to occupational, social and safety problems.

Central Sleep Apnoea

Central sleep apnoea is much less common than OSA. In both conditions the person stops breathing during sleep. However, in central sleep apnoea, the stopping of breathing is due to malfunctioning of the brain centres which coordinate breathing effort.

Central sleep apnoea is seen in people with severe heart problems and in patients with neurological diseases (e.g. strokes). It can be seen in people with no obvious other abnormalities. For example, it can be seen in people living at high altitudes.

Symptoms: Symptoms are similar to OSA, due to sleep fragmentation and lack of oxygen. However, some patients with central sleep apnoea may have no symptoms at all and the diagnosis is made during investigation for other suspected sleep disorders.

Management

Management can be surgical or non-surgical.

Non-surgical management of OSA: Every patient with symptomatic snoring or OSA should be advised various self-help methods which go a long way even after the surgery, for long-term success rates.

Conservative treatment starts with advising various self-help methods, like medical management with drugs which have a respiratory stimulant action and discontinue drugs which have a depressant action on CNS. The other lines of management are intranasal drops, intraoral devices and CPAP.

Self-help methods: After going over various aspects of snoring, there remains little doubt that snoring or OSA goes along with morbid obesity. So, the first approach to treatment for majority of patients is a planned weight reduction programme.

Obesity

The ideal weights may be obtained from the tables made as per age, sex, height and weight of individuals. Obesity is at least 20% more than ideal weight and morbid obesity is about 45 kg above ideal weight.

Since obesity or excess body weight takes the shape of fat and the pattern of distribution of this excess fat, especially in the neck areas induces obstruction to the free airflow. Also, the excess body weight and fat lead to dependant airway obstruction. It is interesting to note that obese men have more fat distribution in their necks inducing snoring when compared to morbidly obese premenopausal women. Reason could be due to hormonal factors.

Another factor causing snoring in obese individuals is reduced stimulation of nerves to the genioglossus muscle thus inducing OSA.

Management of obesity: Apart from a strict diet control, stress is to be placed on regular exercises which improve the tone of muscles and help the airway to be open.

Role of alcohol: Another important thing in the self-help methods is restricting alcohol consumption. Apart from being important co-existing factor in obesity, alcohol acts as depressant, increasing the frequency of disordered breathing and increasing oxygen desaturation.

Change in posture: Partners of the patients or the third party often have noticed that they can sleep better when the patient sleeps on his/her side. They often devise a lot of improvisations to achieve this, like strapping a ball or a marble on the back which makes the patients inconvenient to sleep supine.

Drugs: It is important that patients with OSA avoid using drugs that depress CNS, like the sleeping pills or alcohol. Drugs which relieve nasal congestion like nasal drops and decongestants can be used.

Tricyclic antidepressants like protryptiline, Aminotryptiline are advised which act by decreasing the frequency of more severe REM-related aponea.

Respiratory stimulants like acetolamide, progesterone, theophylline can be tried with a caution.

Thyroid supplements in thyroid deficient patients are to be used.

Devices

1. A ball tied to the back, as already described.
2. Nasal trumpets: A device similar to nasal airway used by anaesthetist to keep the airflow free.
3. Intranasal splints and adhesive straps to achieve the nasal flare.
4. MRA (Mandible repositioning appliance): Is custom made designed to keep the mandible in a forward position thereby positioning the tongue anteriorly and increasing the upper airway size.

Continuous positive air pressure (CPAP)

A lot of patients do get benefit by using this apparatus. In this, oxygen/air are pumped at 5-15 cm of H_2O pressure, continuously through a facial/nasal mask to open up the obstructed airway as well as maintaining higher O_2 saturation which prevents apnoeic episodes. The problem of tolerance to this must be considered. The drawbacks may range from poor compliance with wearing a mask, continuous noise, dry mouth, rhinorrhoea, conjunctivitis, headache, inflammatory facial reactions.

Mandibular Repositioning Appliance

Mandibular repositioning appliance (MRA) is designed to posture the mandible in a forward position thereby respositioning the tongue anteriorly and increasing the upper airway size.

The MRA, a modification of frankels appliance, is basically constructed of heat cured acrylic pads—two buccal pads on each side, two mental pads and one floor mouth pad held together by stainless steel wires. The appliance obtains anchorage to the maxilla and when in position results in protrusion of the mandible.

This appliance is custom made for each patient after taking the dental impression of the upper and lower teeth. This is so constructed as to give about 50% of the maximum protrusion the patient is capable of.

Surgical Management

In 1964, Kematsu described a surgical procedure to correct snoring. But it was Fujita's modification of this procedure that revolutionised surgical treatment modalities. The uvulopalatopharyngoplasty (UPPP) was utilised to reduce the degree of pharyngeal obstruction by removing the redundant tissue in the posterior pharynx and soft palate as well as the tonsillar pillars. Even though this procedure has been modified by various surgeons, it continues to be the most commonly performed surgery for OSA.

As more has been learned about the role of the tongue base, the tongue mass and the lower jaw, attention was focussed on management of obstruction at this site. Even though UPPP has proved to be an excellent surgical procedure for obstruction at the velopharyngeal level, it has limited use when other levels are affected. This results in relatively poor results in patients where UPPP is used as the only treatment modality. Simmons et al concluded that UPPP was highly successful in control of snoring but was successful in only 50% of patients in alleviating OSA. Robert W. Riley et al reviewed unsuccessful UPPP procedures and concluded that the base of the tongue was the cause of persistent obstruction. Riley et al reported success rates of around 80% in controlling snoring and excessive daytime somnolance (EDSD) when all levels were treated.

As any obstruction in the upper airway could be the cause of snoring and OSA, it is realistic to expect that all levels of obstruction should be treated to achieve good results.

UPPP

The area of the velopharyngeal sphincter forms the most common site of obstruction in snoring and OSA and is almost always involved. As such, UPPP forms the mainstay of surgical treatment. This surgical procedure, made popular by Fujita, has undergone modifications by several surgeons. It basically involves excision of the tonsils (if they have not been removed already), the uvula and excess soft tissue of the soft palate, avoiding injury to particularly the posterior pillar and musculature of the soft palate. The pillars and edges of the soft palate are sutured together using vicryl. This procedure not only reduces the bulk of the vibrating soft palate but also increases the distance between the soft palate and the posterior pharyngeal wall and increases the size of the sphincter.

Injury to the posterior pillar could result in velopharyngeal stenosis and excision of the palatal musculature could cause velopharyngeal incompetence. This procedure can be combined with simultaneous surgical treatment of other areas, e.g. septoplasty, turbinectomy, tongue base advancement, etc.

Laser-assisted Uvulopalatoplasty (LAUP)

This procedure was largely popularised by Kamami and is aimed at reducing the size of the uvula and soft palate using laser. Its main advantage is that it can be done as an OP procedure under LA.

The short-term success rates have been reported to be good in controlling snoring although long-term studies have been less satisfying.

Diathermy-assisted Uvulopalatoplasty (DAUP)

It is similar to LAUP but instead of laser handpiece, a fine microdissection diathermy needle is used.

Somnoplasty

Somnoplasty system is designed to use radiofrequency (RF) energy to provide a minimally invasive and less painful treatment for upper airway obstructions under LA. The procedure is performed on an outpatient basis. The patients can return to their normal activities the following day. More than one procedure is necessary to achieve optimal results. This procedure effectively treats OSA by shrinking the base of the tongue—the most difficult source of obstruction to treat in moderately and severely effected patients.

Surgery for Tongue Base Obstruction

Island Mandibulotomy and Hyoid Suspension for Tongue Advancement

Using two horizontal skin incisions in the upper neck an island is prepared in the midline of the mandible using cutting burrs and micro-osteotomes. The bony island is brought out so that the posteriorly attached genioglossus muscle is pulled forwards. The hyoid bone is pulled upwards after all the infra-hyoid muscles are cut and then suspended to the mandible using prolene.

Tracheostomy: It is an excellent way to relieve the obstruction and is extremely useful in severe cases of OSA. This may be a temporary procedure and can be reversed after the specific surgeries are done. Sometimes it is permanent, especially in morbidly obese patients. A valved tracheostomy tube is inserted and it is kept open during the sleeping hours and closed when the patient is awake. In our experience, we had to resort to tracheostomy on only two occasions among the 100 cases that went in for surgery. Both cases were subsequently decannulated.

Other procedures like hyoid expansion, advancement palatoplasty, wedge resection of tongue, etc., have been tried by various workers and results are awaited.

CONCLUSION

OSA as a clinical entity has come to stay and we as otolaryngologists will be called upon to play a leading role in the management of this condition. Our experience over the past 8 to 9 years has indicated that this condition is not uncommon in our country. Most of the patients can be managed non-surgically. The small percentage of patients going in for surgery have excellent short-term results. Studies are needed to assess the long-term results.

CHAPTER

9

Surgery for Tracheal Stenosis

Sultan A. Pradhan, Anil K. D'Cruz, Prathamesh S. Pai

INTRODUCTION

The incidence of tracheal stenosis is on the rise. It is a paradox that the expert intensive care that saves lives of critically ill patients has inadvertently, contributed to this rising trend, for, tracheal stenosis is often the complication of tracheal intubation in patients requiring prolonged ventillatory support. There is significant morbidity associated with the condition, patients often having to lead a life with a tracheostomy, which affects both speech and breathing. Fortunately, it is an avoidable complication, provided there is an increased awareness and proper training of personnel who handle critically ill patients with tracheal intubation. A more disciplined approach will go a long way in the prevention of tracheal stenosis. In India, majority of patients of tracheal stenosis are only in their 'teens and twenties'—sequel of a social tragedy amongst youngsters attempting suicide by consumption of organophosphorous compounds and requiring ventillatory support for resuscitation.

ANATOMY

The adult trachea measures 11 cm in length from the inferior border of the cricoid cartilage to the carinal spur. There are 18 to 22 cartilaginous rings in the human trachea, with approximately two rings per centimetre. The rings are C-shaped, connected posteriorly by a membranous portion of the trachea, the only complete cartilaginous structure in the normal airway being the cricoid. Each cartilage is enclosed in a perichondrium, which is continuous with a dense irregular connective tissue forming a fibrous membrane between adjacent rings of cartilage. The fibrous layers of the perichondrium and the fibrous membrane are composed mainly of collagen with some elastin fibres intermingled. These fibres cross each other diagonally allowing changes in the diameter of the enclosed airway and this provides elastic recoil when the membrane is stretched. The blood supply to the tracheal framework comes from a branch of the inferior thyroid artery, which courses downward to supply both the oesophagus and the trachea. The lower trachea is supplied chiefly by the bronchial vessels. The blood supply is largely end-vessel and segmental without any major longitudinal vessels. The blood vessels enter the trachea laterally.

The recurrent laryngeal nerves course along the trachea in close proximity to the tracheo-oesophageal groove. They ascend up to the lower border of the inferior constrictors of the pharynx, pass behind them and the cricothyroid joint, and then pierce the cricothyroid membrane to enter the larynx. This aspect is to be borne in mind to prevent inadvertant damage to the nerve while mobilising the trachea or while excising the scarred segment of cricoid posteriorly.

About half the adult trachea can be resected and end-to-end anastomosis achieved. However, the trachea must be mobilised to achieve tension free anastomosis. The various manoeuvers done for this are :

1. Laryngeal drop — Suprahyoid [Montgomery]
   — Infrahyoid [Dedo]
2. Carinal release
3. Incising the annular ligament.

The larynx is suspended from the hyoid. The hyoid is attached to the mandible and the skull base by the suprahyoid muscles such as the myelohyoid, geniohyoid, the stylohyoid, and the digastic tendon. Releasing the attachments of these muscles from hyoid will result in a laryngeal "drop".

The length of the trachea may be increased by incising the annular membrane on one hemicircumference, preserving the inner mucoperichondrium. Since the blood supply is lateral with no longitudinal vessels the annular ligaments can be incised safely without causing ischaemic damage to the underlying tracheal framework. However, the annular ligament should be incised only on one side of the trachea proximal to the stenosed segment and on the contralateral side in the segment distal to the stenosis. Once the recoil is reduced in the few segments the tension is reduced over the anastomosis.

Aetiology

Tracheal stenosis can be congenital and acquired (Table 9.1). Congenital tracheal stenosis is a very rare disorder characterised by the presence of a variable number of complete cartilaginous tracheal rings resulting in a fixed tracheal narrowing. The management of this condition is out of scope of this chapter.

Table 9.1

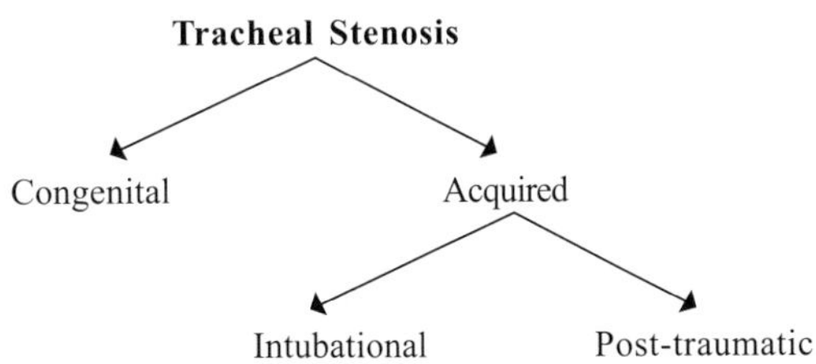

Among the acquired tracheal stenosis the two most common aetiological factors are: intubational injuries and post-traumatic stenosis.

1. *Intubational Injuries*

Intubational injuries are the most common cause of tracheal stenosis. Intubation is frequently necessary to provide ventillatory care to the critically ill. Earlier, if this was necessary for more than 48 hours, a tracheostomy was performed. With the availability of endotracheal tubes of less reactive material (polytetrafluoroethylene) with a low-pressure cuff, clinicians tend to avoid tracheostomy for prolonged periods occasionally as long as 7-10 days.

Prolonged intubation causes ischaemic pressure damage at the level of the inflated cuff of the tube. In case of a tracheostomy the pressure could also occur at the the level of the stoma. The majority of cases in our experience have been post-intubational stenosis.

Pathogenesis: Prolonged intubation produces circumferential pressure injury in the trachea, resulting in ischaemic necrosis. This is very common with high-pressure cuffs. However, a low-pressure cuff when overinflated or used for a prolonged period can have a similar effect.

Improperly suspended heavy equipment coupling the tracheostomy tube to the ventillator can lead to leverage of the tube. This causes erosion of the tracheal wall anteriorly and laterally. Superadded infection further compounds the problem. The result is cicatricial healing of the stoma and stenosis. Since the anterior and lateral wall are eroded, the stenosis is "A" shaped when viewed through a bronchoscope.[1]

Besides the stenosis at the site of the cuff and at the sites of the stoma, damage to the trachea can also be caused at the following sites:

a. The tip of the tracheostomy tube may cause pressure injury to the anterior tracheal wall.
b. Subglottic stenosis may occur if the tracheotomy is placed very high, i.e., close to the cricoid cartilage. The stenosis is then above the stomal site. This is due to chondritis, oedema and scarring.
c. Varying degrees of erosion of cartilages may also occur in the segment between the tracheostome and the level of the cuff due to inflammation. Sometimes the segment may become malacic.
d. The endotracheal tube besides causing a tracheal stenosis (due to overinflated or continuously inflated cuff) may also cause glottic stenosis at the cricoid level. This is of particular importance as corrective surgery on the tracheal stenosis can be disastrous if there is an inadequately functioning glottis above it.

2. *Post-traumatic Stenosis*

Separation of the cervical trachea and blunt injuries to the neck can result in tracheal stenosis. The separation may occur by avulsion of the trachea from the larynx just below the cricoid cartilage or at a lower level. The usual causes of separation or blunt trauma are: a. Vehicular injuries where the neck strikes the edge of the steering wheel or the dash board, b. an accident where the neck is caught by a cable such as motor bike riding or by a '*dupatta*' caught in a table fan or in some such machinery. When primary repair is not done or has failed, strictures result. A long defect will appear to be present since the trachea drops into the mediastinum when it is detached from the larynx. Associated recurrent laryngeal nerve injury is almost always present and compounds the problem.

CLINICAL PRESENTATION AND DIAGNOSIS

History and clinical presentation give the presumptive diagnosis in most cases. Patients with post-intubation stenosis present with signs of upper airway obstruction. Shortness of breath on exertion may soon progress to dyspnoea at rest, wheezing and stridor. Any patient who develops signs of upper airway obstruction must be assumed to have an organic lesion of the trachea, particularly if he has been subjected to intubation at any time in the recent past. In practice, many of these patients have been diagnosed as having adult onset asthma despite the history of recent intubation.

The anteroposterior and lateral neck X-ray studies with the patient's head fully extended are essential to outline the air column of the cervical trachea. Anteroposterior and lateral xeroradiography (which uses charged selenium plates) clearly outline the site, type and degree of stenosis. Fluoroscopy is useful for identifying the tracheomalacia where the segment without support will be seen to collapse during inspiration. CT or MRI scans may be required for additional detail. Laryngoscopy and bronchoscopy help determine the exact level of stenosis by allowing the surgeon to visualise such known landmarks as the vocal cords and the tracheostomy orifice. In patients with an impaired airway without a tracheostomy, endoscopy is preferred until definitive surgery is planned to avoid precipitating acute airway obstruction. It is mandatory to assess the entire length of the trachea before a treatment decision. It is not uncommon to find a stenosis at more than one level.

PREVENTION OF TRACHEAL STENOSIS

The most important measures for prevention of tracheal stenosis start in the intensive care units and in the emergency rooms, where access to the trachea is often required to establish an airway for tracheo-bronchial toilet or to provide ventillatory support.

A lot has gone into the design of endotracheal and tracheostomy tubes such as use of less reactive material and low-pressure cuffs with shapes that distribute the pressure evenly over a larger area, thus minimising pressure necrosis. However, there is no short cut to a certain discipline that needs to be followed by the staff of the intensive care unit. It is important to emphasise the following:

- Even tubes with low-pressure cuffs can be dangerous when overinflated. The golden rule to avoid complicaton is to strictly keep the cuff deflated when possible or alternatively to adhere strictly to the practise of deflating the cuff for 3-5 minutes every hour.
- When an endotracheal tube is kept post-operatively only to maintain an airway and not for positive pressure ventillatory support, there is generally no need to keep the cuff inflated.
- A high tracheostomy should be avoided. When a tracheostomy is placed just below the cricoid cartilage, it can result in subglottic and upper tracheal oedema and subsequent stenosis. If a high tracheostomy is already existent, it should be revised by performing a lower fenestration and the patient should be treated with systemic steroids and antibiotics.
- An elective tracheostomy should be performed under ideal conditions and not be hurried. The opening in the trachea should be at the level of the third ring or below for reasons mentioned above.
- Care must be taken to see that the tubes connecting the tracheostomy tube to the ventillator are properly supported to prevent any tilt or angulation of the tracheostomy tube. Such a tilt may cause the tube to erode back into the upper tracheal rings and the cricoid leading to ulceration, oedema and subsequently stenosis.
- Infection at the tracheostomy site is best prevented by the use of sterile suction catheters, frequent change of the entire tube, and regular dressings. If, however, infection does set in, it should be recognised and treated promptly with appropriate antibiotics since infection contributes greatly to stenosis.

- An obstruction of the trachea at the end of the tracheostomy tube should be suspected when the patient complains of intermittent respiratory difficulty and the necessity for frequent adjustment of the tracheostomy tube. An immediate by-pass of the area by inserting an endotracheal tube may be life saving.
- After the tracheostomy has been removed if there are any symptoms of impaired airway, the trachea should be immediately evaluated with lateral neck X-rays, laminagraphy or computerised imaging. A tracheoscopy should not be deferred if there is any question of stenosis.

TREATMENT OF TRACHEAL STENOSIS

Treatment of Acute Tracheal Stenosis

In acute tracheal stenosis, there is mainly oedema and granulation, which cause the stenosis. Fibrosis has not yet set in. Granulomas in the subglottic region interfering with the airway are resected endoscopically with the carbon dioxide (CO_2) laser coupled to the operating microscope. A steroid injection into the site of the origin of the granuloma is useful in preventing a recurrence. If a high tracheotomy has been the cause of the subglottic oedema and granulations, it is revised and placed at a lower level.

Stenosis of the lower cervical or upper thoracic trachea, occurring at the site of the tip of the tracheostomy tube or the endotracheal tube can create an acute emergency. As a first step, an endotracheal tube or a longer tracheostomy tube is inserted to go beyond the obstruction. Once the emergency is taken care of, the granuloma is resected endoscopically through a tracheoscope or a bronchoscope coupled to the CO_2 laser. The procedure may need to be repeated until the healing is complete. In the interim period, the region is stented with the use of a silicon tracheostomy T-tube. A steriod injection in the base of the granuloma is advocated to prevent fibrosis. All possible measures should be taken to prevent a fibrous stricture at this site, since segmental resection at this level carries a significant morbidity.

If an acute airway problem is the result of a crushing injury to the tracheal cartilaginous rings, open reduction and stenting with a silicon tube is the treatment of choice. This allows maintenance of the tracheal lumen while the cartilages heal in the correct anatomic position.

Treatment of Chronic Tracheal Stenosis

In this type of stenosis there is damage to the tracheal framework and fibrosis has already set in.

1. *Stenosis following Endotracheal Tube Injury*

Endotracheal tubes can cause tracheal stenosis either at the site of the cuff of the tube and/or at the site of the tip of the tube. Before discussing the treatment of stenosis at these sites it is important to reiterate that endotracheal tubes being translaryngeal, may also cause damage to the larynx leading to oedema, granulations or even web formation. These if present should be attended to prior to undertaking repair of the tracheal stenosis.

a. *Treatment for stenosis at the site of the cuff*: These are circumferential stenosis of the trachea, with loss of mucosal continuity. The extent of the cartilage damage varies and is generally not so severe as in the case of a tracheostomy tube injury, because the infective element is less. If the cartilaginous framework is maintained, these strictures will respond to repeated dilatations, assisted when necessary, with sharp release incision with the CO_2 laser, endoscopically.

If stenosis is a tight or if the stenosed segment is longer than a centimetre, making release incisions with CO_2 laser becomes difficult and repeated, failed attempts would worsen the stenosis due to charring. In these situations in adults (age more than 18 years) a permanent, self-expanding metallic stent can be placed, provided there is at least a 4 mm lumen to allow its introduction. In younger individuals (age less than 18 years) or in adults where the lumen is very narrow and a guidewire cannot be negotiated through the stenosis, resection with end-to-end anastomosis is the treatment of choice.

b. *Treatment of tracheal stenosis at the site of tip of the endotracheal tube*: These stenoses are at or beyond the thoracic inlet. Resection and end-to-end anastomosis carries a high mortality rate and is, therefore, to be avoided as far as possible. The treatment of choice in adults is endoscopic stenting with the permanent self-expanding metallic tube. In children dilatation and temporary stenting is performed, using a silicon tracheostomy T-tube.

2. *Stenosis following Tracheotomy Intubation*

Tracheal stenosis following prolonged intubation through a tracheotomy can occur at four sites:

A. At the stoma level
B. Above the stoma
C. Below the stoma
 — At the site of the cuff
 — At the site of the tip of the tracheostomy tube

A. *Treatment for Stenosis at the Site of the Stoma*: This is a common site for developing stenosis. Either, there is a buckling in, or necrosis of the tracheal cartilage at the level of the tracheostome leading to stenosis.

i. *Buckling-in deformity of the tracheal rings*: Traumatic and hurried tracheotomy with a H-shaped incision results in buckling of the rings. This needs 'release' incisions over the fibrotic area and stenting of the lumen with a silastic T-tube. The anterior segment can also be excised and repaired using the sternohyoid muscle and fascia.[11]

ii. *Cartilage necrosis*: Where there is loss of two or three tracheal rings anteriorly, and the posterior mucosa is intact, a wedge resection can be performed with direct closure of the defect. A sterno-mental stitch [Freedmans Procedure] is advisable for a period of 10 days to avoid tension on the repair. However, when the circumferential damage is >50% or if a longer segment of the trachea is involved, the treatment of choice is resection and end-to-end anastomosis.

B. Treatment for Stenosis above the Stoma

i. *Buckling-in deformity of the tracheal rings:* A traumatic tracheostomy can result in buckling of the anterior tracheal wall above the tracheostome. The tracheostome is revised and placed as inferiorly as possible. The tracheal rings have now to be upturned into their natural position. The buckled cartilages are incised vertically in the midline. Additional vertical incisions are required if there is extensive fibrosis keeping the inner perichondrium intact, to 'release' the buckled rings to their normal anatomic position. The trachea is then stented with a silicon T-tube. The T-tube is plugged to avoid dehydration of the tracheal stenosis and to avoid frequent suctioning and the resultant trauma to the trachea. This allows the patient to breathe and speak normally. The T-tube can be removed after 6 to 8 weeks.

ii. *Cartilage necrosis*:

a. *Loss of anterior tracheal support*: Loss of the anterior portion of one or more rings of the tracheal cartilage above the tracheostomy site results in collapse of the lateral walls, resulting in a slit-like scar. The tracheostomy is revised and placed as inferiorly as possible. An anterior midline vertical incision is made in the scarred collapsed segment. Fibrous and granulation tissues are resected and the lateral walls are retracted with skin hooks. A silicon T-tube is inserted and the anterior tracheal wall is reconstructed with the strap muscles sutured over it. The T-tube is then plugged for the reasons described above and is removed after 6 to 8 weeks.

b. *Circumferential stenosis*: These are a result of a high tracheotomy performed at the level of the first and second tracheal rings. These are complex stenoses involving not only the upper cervical trachea but also the lower subglottic region. These are extremely difficult to treat and pose a challenge to the skills of the treating physician. Resection anastomosis is treatment of choice, is technically very demanding and the results are not good.

C. *Treatment for Stenosis below the Stoma*

i. *Treatment for stenosis at the site of the 'cuff'*: Whether the 'cuff' of a tracheostomy tube causes stenosis or the cuff of an endotracheal tube causes it, the management is essentially the same and is discussed in the earlier section. However, patients receiving ventillatory support through a tracheostomy tube have had ventillatory support for longer period of time than those intubated with an endotracheal tube. Consequently, the damage to the cartilagenous framework is more. This is further compounded with the infective element from an open tracheostomy wound. These stenoses are, therefore, rarely amenable to simpler measures of endoscopic CO_2 laser release of stenosis followed by dilatation and stenting. Sleeve resection and anastomosis is generally the treatment of choice. The tracheostome needs to be included in the resected segment and hence very good mobilisation, including a "laryngeal drop" is mandatory, to ensure a tension free anastomosis. The larynx, however, is normal unlike in the case of endotracheal tube injury.

ii. *Treatment for stenosis at the site of "tip" of the tracheostomy tube*: This again is similar to the stenosis caused by the endotracheal tube injury and is discussed earlier.

Treatment of Post-traumatic Stenosis

Post-traumatic stenosis occurs when the avulsed trachea following blunt trauma has not been repaired or when the repair has failed. The most important aspect in managing this type of stenosis is the assessment of the glottis and injury to surrounding structures. The laryngeal framework and the function of the vocal cords need careful evaluation. Tracheo-oesophageal fistulas also have to be looked for.

If the glottis is competent and the larynx is normal, tracheal anastomosis is undertaken. The tracheal remnants are carefully dissected of the oesophagus and a tension free anastomosis is carried out after adequate mobilisation. If required, strap muscles can be sutured on to the oesophagus to prevent a TO fistula.

If the vocal cords are paralysed, procedures are undertaken to achieve a competent and functional glottis and then the tracheal stenosis is tackled as above.

If the laryngeal framework is damaged, then the larynx has to be repaired at the same sitting as the tracheal repair.

Associated Factors

1. *Multiple Stenoses*

At times tracheal stenosis is present at more than one of the four sites mentioned earlier viz., subglottic, stomal site, site of the cuff or at the tip of the tube. If the intervening distance is large, then resection of both strictures in a single segment is hazardous, because it may then not be possible to approximate the two ends without tension. If the two segments are resected individually, the intervening tracheal segment may have a compromised blood supply.

In such a situation a staged approach is recommended.[7] The proximal stenosis is resected first and the distal stenosis which is generally at the level of the thoracic inlet is treated subsequently with endoscopic stenting with self-expandable metallic stents in adults and silicon T-tubes in children.

2. *Paralysed Larynx*

Evaluation of a patient with tracheal stenosis is incomplete without assessing the larynx. In cases of external trauma, recurrent laryngeal nerve injury is always a distinct possibility.

In cases of bilateral cord paralysis with cords in adduction, the patient will have a good voice with occlusion of the tracheotoma. Failure to diagnose this preoperatively will be embarrassing following a successful sleeve resection. There will be a perfect tracheal lumen but an inadequate laryngeal aditus.

In cases of bilateral cord paralysis with the cords in abduction, the laryngeal competence is affected. Failure to diagnose this will be disastrous. The patient will be unable to phonate and will aspirate. There will be a greater disability than with the stenosed trachea.

Every patient of laryngotracheal stenosis should have a mandatory evaluation of the vocal cord function. In case of bilateral vocal paralysis following trauma, at least 6 months have to be given for laryngeal function to possibly return. Electrodiagnostic studies of nerve muscle conduction may be a better objective prognostic indicator.

After observing for 6 to 12 months, without return of laryngeal function, the glottic airway has to established first by appropriate procedures such as cord lateralisation, posterior cordectomy + arytenoidectomy, lateral arytenoidopexy in case of abductor cord palsy (cords in paramedian position) or reverse arytenoidopexy in cases of adductor cord palsy (cords in cadaveric position).

The tracheal stenosis needs evaluation after the glottis has been treated to prevent an incompetent larynx.

SURGICAL TECHNIQUES OF RESECTION ANASTOMOSIS

A. Mid or Lower Cervical Tracheal Resection and Anastomosis

These are simple stenoses not associated with subglottic involvement and hence easier to resect, mobilise and anastomose with very good results.

A collar incision is generally sufficient for access though rarely a median sternotomy may be required if the stenosis involves the lower trachea. The stenotic segment if not easily localised can be identified using a fibreoptic bronchoscope. The trachea is dissected circumferentially around the stenosed segment, keeping close to the trachea to avoid damage to the recurrent laryngeal nerves, and for a distance not more than 1-2 cm proximal and distal to avoid devascularising the portion of trachea that will be used for reconstruction.

Division of the trachea is commenced in a conservative fashion. The final division must be where the mucosa is normal and good cartilaginous rings are present. The stenosed segment is carefully separated from the oesophagus after inspecting it for injury. Proximal and distal traction sutures are placed on the lateral walls. The patients' neck is flexed and the two segments are approximated to ensure that the anastomosis is tension free.

In cases where the two ends cannot be approximated or there is tension, any of the release procedures are undetaken.

Release Techniques

1. *Laryngeal Drop*[2]: This involves release of the larynx from its attachments to the hyoid bone, either superior or inferior to the hyoid. Either technique provides mobilisation up to 5 cm of trachea. The suprahyoid technique is preferred as it is less traumatic and does not interfere with the deglutition process.

   In the *suprahyoid release* technique, suprahyoid strap muscles are detached via a subperichondrial dissection till the greater cornua. The superior laryngeal pedicles lie distal to the greater cornuae of the hyoid. Hence, to avoid damaging them a bone cutter is used to separate the body of the hyoid from the greater cornuae releasing the larynx. The other landmark is to stay medial to the anterior tendon of the digastric muscle.

   In the *infra-hyoid release* technique, the infra-hyoid straps are separated from the hyoid. The thyrohyoid muscles are identified and divided at the superior border of the thyroid cartilage. The superior cornuae of the thyroid are exposed and divided carefully. To avoid injury to the superior laryngeal pedicle, the dissection is kept close to the thyroid cartilage superior border. Finally, the thyrohyoid membrane is divided.
2. *Incising Annular Ligament*[3]: Annular ligaments above and below the site of anastomosis can be sectioned up to the mucosa. This gives us about 1.5 cm additional length. The rings on the proximal segment are divided on side contralateral to the side where the rings are divided on the distal segment. This not only lengthens but also more importantly preserves the vascularity of the trachea.
3. *Grillo's Procedure*[4,5]: This is a method of superior mobilisation of the distal trachea from the thorax. It involves a thoracotomy, followed by mobilisation of the right hilus and division of the pulmonary ligament. The pulmonary vessels are freed from the pericardium. Finally, the left main bronchus is sectioned distal to the carina and reattached to the tracheobronchial system by end-to-end anastomosis with the right main bronchus. This method gives 6 cm of additional length

Once the trachea is mobilised and the release performed to achieve tension free approximation, the closure is begun. The suture material preferred is an absorbable suture preferably Vicryl or Dexon 2-0. The first suture is placed in the midline posteriorly such that the knot lies outside the trachea to prevent subsequent granulation tissue. The sutures are placed approximately 4 mm from the cut edge of the trachea and passed through the full thickness of the tracheal wall. The sutures are then placed but not tied in a series lateral to the first suture until the enitre circumference of the trachea is covered.

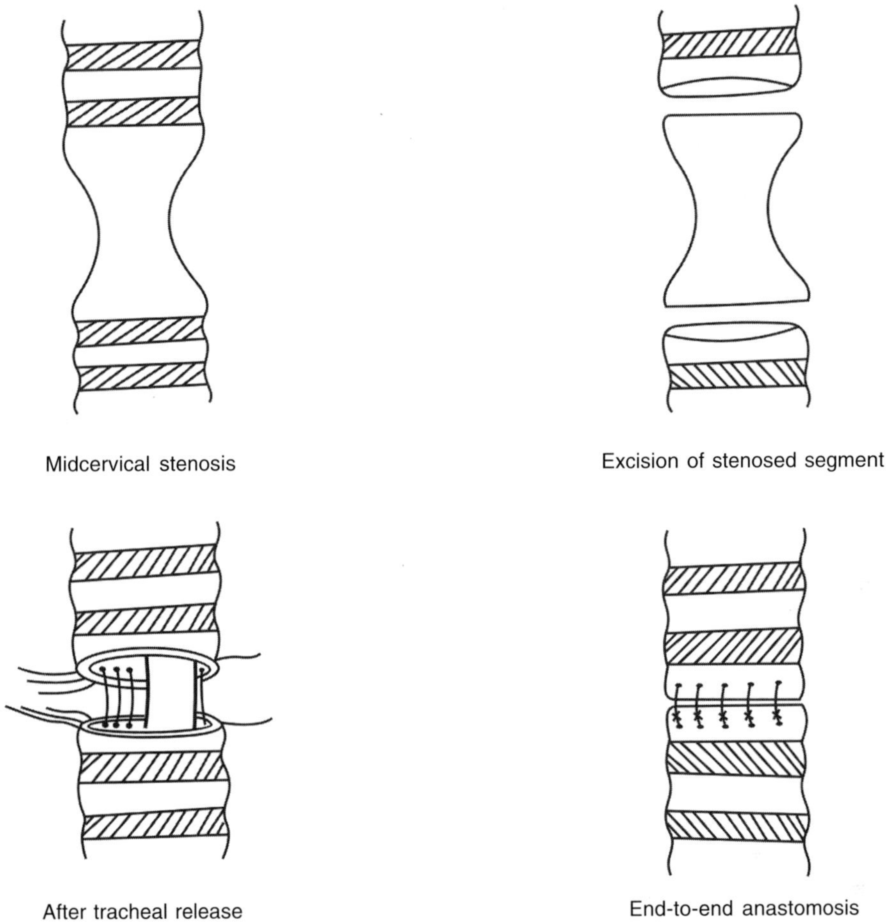

Fig. 9.1: Steps of cervical tracheal resection and anastomosis

The endotracheal tube is then advanced and the lateral traction sutures are tied. Starting anteriorly each individual suture is tied. The anastomosis is assessed after flooding the tracheal bed with saline and ventillating with the endotracheal cuff inflated to check for any obvious leak.

The thyroid isthmus that was divided at the time of mobilisation is approximated. Suction drains are placed and the wound is closed in layers. A sternomental stitch with 1-0 prolene ensures neck flexion. This is kept in place for 5-7 days. The patient is extubated the next day.

B. Subglottic and Upper Tracheal Resection Anastomosis

In the subglottis the stenosis is predominantly anterolateral. The resection involves the anterior part of the cricoid cartilage along with the stenotic tracheal segment. The resection of the cricoid segment begins in the midline at the cricothryroid membrane and then proceeds laterally and inferiorly across the cricothyroid membrane on either side till the superolateral border of the cricoid is reached. The resection continues with the edge levelled downwards and backwards

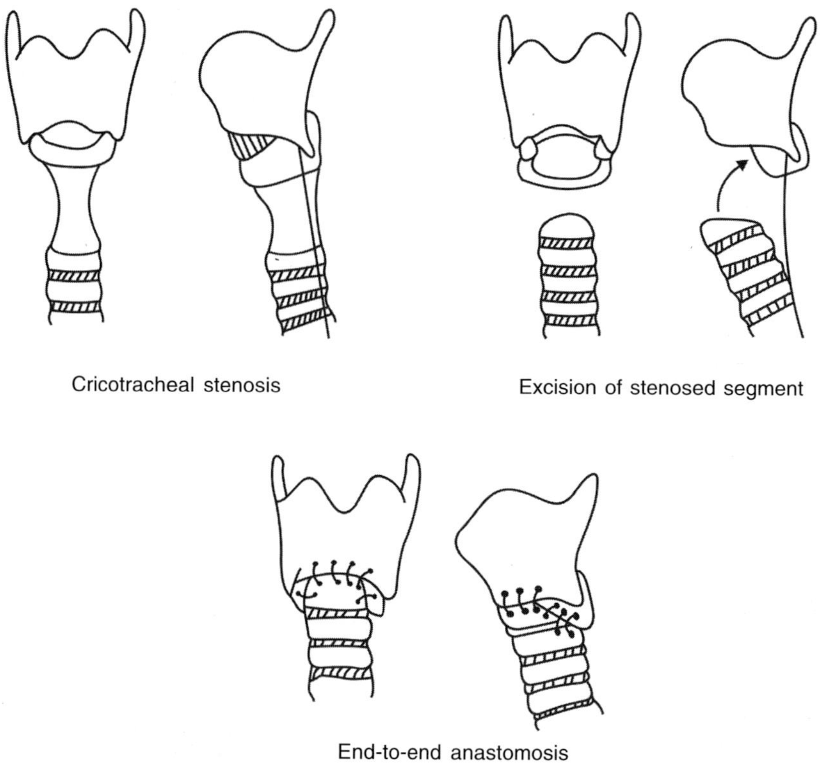

Fig. 9.2: Steps of cricotracheal resection and anastomosis

along the inferior border of the posterior cricoid plate. Care must be taken to avoid damaging the recurrent laryngeal nerves during the complete mucosal transection. The distal end of the trachea is fashioned to conform to the curvature of the proximal resection. This avoids a sharp angulation. The anastomosis is performed as described above for cervical tracheal stenosis between the trachea and the thyroid cartilage anteriorly and the cricoid cartilage posteriorly.[6] A lower tracheostomy may be required to allow the subglottic oedema to settle. The site of the tracheostomy has to be carefully planned to prevent damage to the anastomosis above and to the innominate artery below.

Post-operative Care following Tracheal Resection

Nursing Care

In the post-operative period the patient needs to be nursed with neck in gentle flexion so as to prevent tension on the anastomosis. The patient often needs careful throat suctioning from time to time to prevent aspiration. Heavy sedation must be avoided, keeping in mind the tendency toward aspiration particularly if a laryngeal drop has been performed.

Care of the Airway

The airway needs special attention. If the patient is wide awake in the immediate post-operative period and the anastomosis is satisfactory, he may be extubated in the operating room and observed carefully for any signs of respiratory distress. If these develop, immediate re-intubation is undertaken with extreme caution using a small size tube. A small endotracheal tube is retained across the anastomosis overnight if there is any doubt about the patency of the lumen or if there is an associated factor like cord palsy. The patient is then extubated the following day. Another approach is to do distal tracheostomy, but we do not recommend this. This is done only if there are serious concerns regarding the lumen of the trachea, at the time of anastomosis.

Post-operative Feeding

Ryle's tube feeding is continued for about 5 to 7 days and once the patient is able to accept oral feeds without any aspiration the Ryle's tube is removed.

Complications

- Acute airway obstruction
- Haemorrhage
- Recurrence of stenosis
- Rec. laryngeal nerve injury
- Suture granuloma at the anastomotic site.
- Anastomotic dehiscence.

Acute Airway Obstruction

Occurs if the stenosed segment of the trachea has not been adequately resected, especially in complex stenosis, or there is oedema at the site of the anastomosis, or if there is an associated glottic paralysis. The obstruction should be promptly relieved by passing a small endotracheal tube beyond the obstruction or by performing a tracheostomy, distal to the obstruction. The subsequent treatment depends upon the cause of the obstruction.

Haemorrhage

When the anastomosis is very low (at the thoracic inlet), it is in very close proximity to the innominate artery. This can result in haemorrhage from the innominate artery. It can be prevented by minimum dissection of the artery and by covering the artery with strap muscles.

Damage to the Recurrent Laryngeal Nerve

Damage to the recurrent laryngeal nerve can compromise the airway that may lead to aspiration and result in hoarseness. Dissecting close to the tracheal wall can prevent its damage.

Anastomotic Dehiscence

This is generally a result of excessive tension on the anastomotic suture line, when too much of trachea has been resected or when tracheal or laryngeal release manoeuvres have not been carried out.

Suture Granulomas

Once a very common occurrence, these are rarely seen today due to improved absorbable suture materials.

Recurrence of Stenosis

Granulation or partial dehiscence followed by healing with fibrosis can lead to recurrence of stenosis. With proper case selection and meticulous technique, these can be minimised.

Role of Lasers

Carbon dioxide laser coupled to an operating micsoscope has been used in laryngeal and tracheal stenosis as a precision cutting tool. The laryngeal webs occurring posteriorly, can be released endoscopically without injury to surrounding structures. Within the trachea, the stenotic segment can be widened using radial incisions at 3 different positions.[8,9] The increased lumen so achieved will need to be maintained, either with repeated dilatations for a certain period, or planning a stent until the healing is complete. If this is not done, there will be more scarring with resultant stenosis which is even more severe.

It is important to understand also the limitations of the CO_2 laser in the treatment of stenosis. In cases with loss of cartilaginous support and circumferential stenosis of greater than a centimetre, the carbon dioxide laser has no role. Repeated attempts at laserisation to achieve an adequate airway may be unsuccessful and may even worsen the stenosis due charring and subsequent healing with fibrosis. Such cases need sleeve resection with end-to-end anastomosis.

Stents

Stents are commonly used to support and stabilise reconstructed sites (with grafts or flaps) against mechanical disruption during movements of laryngotracheal complex. They are also used to act as a scaffolding for epithelial coverage of the lumen and to prevent buildup of granulation tissue and subsequent scarring during healing.[10]

Silicon T-tubes

Silicon[11] initiates little or no tissue reaction. It does not change with body temperature nor do body secretions affect it. Hence, it is an ideal material for use as an intratracheal stent which may have to be kept for several weeks or even months, as the trachea heals.

The T-tube has an intraluminal portion which is sufficiently dense and thick to support a reconstituted trachea or a reconstructed trachea and at the same time is soft enough not to injure the lining or supporting structure of the trachea. Ridges and grooves constructed on the extraluminal portion of the T-tube to allow a ring washer attachment to prevent displacement. A speaking valve can also be fitted on to the grooves. The T-tube is supplied in sizes 10 mm, 12 mm, 13 mm and 14 mm (outer diameter). A plug is supplied with the T-tube which when twisted into place occludes the extraluminal part.

Indications

1. Acute tracheal injuries
2. To support a reconstituted trachea
3. To support a reconstructed trachea
4. To support intrathoracic tracheal stenosis
5. Tracheal stenosis when the cervical or thoracic trachea cannot be repaired.

Insertion

The T-tube is generally inserted under general anaesthesia. It can be inserted at the bedside of a patient who has had a T-tube for several months. The end of the intraluminal portion of the T-tube, which is to be inserted inferiorly is folded on itself and grasped with a haemostat. It is then directed into the distal trachea till the entire intraluminal protion is within the trachea. The extraluminal part is the grasped and tugged so ensure proper placement of the upper limb of the T-tube. A ring washer is then applied to the groove adjacent to the skin surface and the groove is marked.

Special Features

The external portion of the T-tube can be tilted superiorly or inferiorly to facilitate suctioning. To prevent loss of anaesthetic agent during surgery an embolectomy catheter with a inflatable balloon is introduced into the upper segment to prevent escape of the gases.

Post-operative Care

Although mucus and crusts do not usually adhere to the smooth walls of the T-tube proper suction is essential initially. Humidification and mucolytic agents such as bromhexine, acetyl cysteine and guafeniscein are important. Care of the external skin is very important. Early diagnosis of secondary infection will prevent granulation and fibrosis.

Self-expandable Metallic Stent (SEMS)

Stents have been used since a long time in maintaining the tracheal lumen. Endoluminal stent placement offers a rapid and effective means of opening up narrowed airways, and results in excellent relief of symptoms and improvement in pulmonary function. For a very long time, the only available stents were the rigid variety made of silicon. They had many drawbacks such as difficulty in introduction, lack of postplacement expansion, lack of complete luminal mucosalisation, and inability to conform to the natural curvature of the trachea. These lead to migration of the stent and retention of secretions, which required frequent bronchoscopic clearance.

Then came the expandable stents made of stainless steel, tantalum, copper alloy, etc. These were designed to reduce migration, but they too had many drawbacks. These had to be expanded with balloon dilatation or had intrinsic elasticity. These also expanded to a predetermined diameter. In either case, there was mucosal damage while introducing or adjusting the stent causing web formation and stenosis at the proximal and distal end, thus defeating their purpose. In addition, the meshwork caused formation of granulation and in some cases erosion of the tracheal wall and adjacent vascular structures.

Recent advances in biomaterials have lead to the discovery of 'superelastic' materials with 'shape memory'. One of these is nickel titanium alloy—**nitinol,** which is biocompatible. It has an ability to undergo large elastic deformity due to a definite inflection point. Such an inflection point in the unloading of coiled nitinol implies the presence of an unloading plateau with near constant stress. Thus, a compact coiled system can be delivered conveniently to a small cross-sectional area and released to expand uniformly throughout its length and circumference. It is, however, important to realise that the nitinol stenting system has no significant capacity to dilate a stenosis. Thus, a dilatation of the stenotic segment and even a laser resection of a fibrotic band need to be done prior to placement of the stent to achieve a proper lumen. Because they are delivered in a nonexpanded state using flexible over-wire systems, they can be placed using a flexible bronchoscope. The stents epithelialise, which prevents migration and permits ciliary activity to continue.

Prior to the pacement of any of these SEMS, computed tomography is essential in imaging, as it allows:

1. Accurate representation of airway anatomy in three dimensions,
2. Measurement of airway diameter,
3. Evaluation of airway anatomy distal to a narrowed segment and invisible to bronchoscopy,
4. Demonstration of dynamic changes in airway morphologic features during forced exhalation in patients with airway tracheomalacia, and
5. Demonstration of, focal or diffuse air trapping in lung peripheral to the abnormal airway.

In patients who have had stent placement, computed tomography is valuable in assessing airway morphologic features and dynamics distal to the stent, and can be valuable in assessing stent dysfunction.

Indications

Tracheo-bronchial stenoses produced by malignant neoplasms or in benign stenosis.

Contraindications

1. SEMS should not be used in tracheo-oesophageal fistulae unless they have inner sheathing.
2. The lumen should be at least 4 mm in order to facilitate the stent placement.

Stent Placement

The procedure can be performed under local anaesthesia or general anaesthesia using either intermittent ventillation or jet ventillation via the suspension laryngoscope. Flexible bronchoscope is used to visualise the stenotic segment, which is dilated.[12] If there is a thick fibrous band, laser resection or radial cuts are used to release the stenosis. The lumen is dilated to approximately to that of the proximal normal tracheal lumen.

The length of the stenosed segment is now measured from the distal end to the proximal end. This is done using a bronchoscope. The stent has to be properly selected. The length of the stent should be at least 10 to 20 mm more so that it can overlap the normal mucosa on either side. The diameter should be approximately the size of the normal proximal tracheal lumen. Most adults require stents with 18 to 20 mm diameter.[13]

The stent can be deployed under flouroscopic control or under vision using the flexible bronchoscope. Under fluoroscopy the radio-opaque markers are visualised and positioned such that the stricture is centralised and then the stent is deployed gently.

Using the flexible bronchoscope the guidewire is introduced beyond the distal end of the stenosis. The stent is then advanced over the guidewire such that the distal end of the stent is beyond the stenosed end and then the bronchoscope is withdrawn above the proximal end of the stent. The stent is then deployed gently.

Complications

Although the procedure is simple, stent placement can be associated with various complications such as:

1. Stent misplacement
2. Haemorrhage
3. Tracheal perforation

4. Pneumothorax
5. Stent migration
6. Stent obstruction due to mucus accumulation
7. Tumour ingrowth in malignant strictures, hence sheathed stents preferred
8. Granulations
9. Tracheal ulceration
10. Stent fracture
11. Infection and septic shock.
    Significant complications can occur, but complications that are more serious are uncommon.

CONCLUSIONS

Tracheal stenosis incidence is on the rise. It is totally avoidable with adequate precautions and care. There have been advances in the treatment modalities available, however, it is difficult to treat stenoses involving the larynx, with the chest and multiple complex stenoses. Stents, a recent development, will help reduce the incidence of major surgery. However, whatever the case, the condition and treatment is morbid and results unpredictable. Therefore, meticulous aherence to discipline and education of the ICU staff is essential to avoid this condition.

REFERENCES

1. Grillo HC, Mathisen, DJ. Surgical management of tracheal strictures. Surgical Clinics of North America, 1988; Vol. 68, No.3.
2. Dedo HH and Fishman, NH. Laryngeal release and sleeve resection for tracheal stenosis. Ann. Otol. Rhinol. Laryngol. 1969; 78:285.
3. Som ML. Reconstruction of the larynx and trachea: Report of a case of extensive cicatricial stenosis. J. Mount Sinai Hosp. 1951; 17:1117-26.
4. Grillo HC. Circumferential: Resection and reconstruction of the mediastinal and cervical trachea. Ann. Surg. 1965; 162: 374-88.
5. Barclay RS. McSwam H, Welsh TM: Tracheal reconstruction without the use of grafts. Thorax 1957; 12:177.
6. Grillo HC: Primary reconstruction of airway after resection of subglottic laryngeal and upper tracheal stenosis. Ann. Thorac Surg 1981; 33:3.
7. Biller HF. Lawson W and Weisberg V. Staged repair of extensive tracheal and laryngotracheal stenosis. Ann. Otol Rhinol Laryngol, 1986; 95:586-89.
8. Shapsay SM, Beamis JF, Hybels RL, Bohigan RK. Endoscopic treatment of subglottic and tracheal stenosis by radial laser incision and dilatation. Annals of Otology, Rhinology and Laryngology, 1987; 96: 661-64.
9. Ossof RH, Tucker GF Jr, Duncavage JA. et al: Efficacy of bronchoscopic carbon dioxide laser surgery for benign strictures of trachea, Laryngoscope, 1985; 95:1220-23.
10. Zalzal GH. Use of stents in laryngotracheal reconstruction in children: Indications, technical considerations and complications. Laryngoscope, 1982; 98:849-54.
11. Montgomery W. Surgery of the upper respiratory system, vol. II, Lea and Febiger, 1989.
12. Wilson G, Walshaw MJ, Hind CRK. Treatment of large airway obstruction in lung cancer using expandable metal stents inserted under direct vision via the fibreoptic bronchoscope. Thorax 1996; 52:248-52.
13. Ducic Y, Khalafi RS. Use of endoscopically placed expandable nitinol tracheal stents in the treatment of tracheal stenosis. Laryngoscope, 1999; 109:1130-33.

CHAPTER

10

Inhaled Foreign Bodies

Anil Malhotra, Vinod H Shah

It is quite common for otolaryngologists to encounter foreign bodies in their day-to-day practice. Of all these, the foreign bodies that land in the respiratory tract are the most dangerous and challenging to manage. These foreign bodies not only jeopardize the respiration, but are also difficult to remove because of various reasons:

1. Such foreign bodies are most commonly seen in early childhood and in the initial period, tend to get neglected and undiagnosed unless present in the glottis or subglottis. The baby cannot give a history and there may not be a witness available.
2. When reporting late, they tend to get impacted in the lower regions of bronchi.
3. Many times, the foreign bodies are organic ones like vegetable seeds and nuts (groundnut being the most common), which set up local mucosal inflammation at the site of impaction.
4. The removal has to be done under general anaesthesia, during which the anaesthetist and the endoscopist vie for the same space, which is quite narrow.

Toddlers are more vulnerable because they have a tendency and a curiosity to put things in their mouths, have poor mastication and relatively weaker reflexes during deglutition and they do inadvertently put things in their mouths while playing, crying, laughing or shouting. These babies do initially cough or choke over the foreign bodies but if the cough is not strong enough, the foreign body descends to carina or bronchus. In most of such instances, a chronic situation develops and there are no alarming symptoms. On the other hand, in the cases where the FB impacts in the larynx or subglottis, immediate attention is drawn due to marked stridor. Organic and sharp-edged FBs, when inhaled, produce worse scenarios.

Multiple FBs are rare (Rothman and Boeckman, 1980).[1] If a FB is aspirated in to a bronchus, it is more likely to go to the right bronchus since it has less angulation with the trachea and is slightly wider. These can sometimes be coughed out spontaneously; but even if it so happens, and the patient's condition does not improve significantly, it is necessary to perform an exploratory endoscopy.

Endoscopy for the removal of an inhaled FB is in the province of an otorhinolaryngologist. Nowadays, such removal is usually a controlled, well-monitored and uneventful procedure for an experienced anaesthetist and a surgeon, in contrast to the olden days when modern facilities like cardiac monitor, pulse oxymeter or ventilating bronchoscopes were not available. Removal of an inhaled FB is as much a test of skill of the anaesthetist as of the surgeon. The present safety of endoscopy in children is more due to developments in anaesthesia like constant detailed monitoring of cardiorespiratory functions. Better understanding of pathophysiological status of suffering children and visualization through telescopes with better illumination and convenience of extended time availability has improved the results to a large extent.

Historical Aspects and Advances

The first successful bronchoscopy is credited to Gustav Killian (1897), when he used a 9 mm tube for the purpose. Distal illumination was added by Eihorn in 1902. However, the pioneering work leading to modern day bronchoscopy was done by Chevaliar Jackson in the 1930s, who designed instruments and techniques for safe bronchoscopic removal of FBs. His famous chalk talks and illustrations are the earliest evidence of importance of documentation in the study of this science. He was also responsible for educating the public on the hazards of inhaled FBs and its preventive measures.

His illustrious work was then continued by his students–Jackson Jr., Holinger and Tucker Sr.. The major breakthrough in illumination came with Broyles (1963) demonstrating use of fibreoptic light in endoscopy. Holinger (1965) developed fibreoptic carriers for endoscopes without impingement on the narrow lumen. In 1972, Holinger and Brubaker presented the method of still and motion picture photography through Storz Hopkin's telescope. The advent of Hopkin's rod lens system, described by Ward et. al. (1974)[3] and ventilating bronchoscopes (Hopkins, 1976)[4] ushered in a new era in this field.

Modern pediatric endoscopy owes a great deal to Paul Ward, George Berce, Eigi Yanagigisawa and Bruce Benjamin for their pioneering efforts, teaching methods and excellent documentation.

Anatomical and Physiological Considerations

The glottis of a newborn infant has anteroposterior length of 7 mm and posterior transverse breadth of 4 mm. Hence, even 1 mm of mucosal edema will reduce the space by 35%. The subglottic diameter is 5 mm. At birth, the epiglottis is at 1st cervical vertebra and cricoid at 3rd cervical. There is a gradual descent of larynx to the level of 5th or 6th vertebrae during adult life. The larynx continues to enlarge evenly in males and females till puberty; after which, the male larynx expands more than the female. So, in adult life, the male larynx is 35 mm in sagittal dimension, 43 mm. in coronal plane and 44 mm. deep; while in females, the dimensions are only 25 mm × 41 mm × 35 mm. The cords are 17-19 mm apart posteriorly in full abduction in adults.

The trachea is about 4.2-4.3 cm long at 6-12 months of age and attains its full length of average 12 cm in adulthood. It bifurcates in the adult at the level of the 5th thoracic vertebra into two principle bronchi. A keel like projection, the carina separates the two bronchi.

The right principle bronchus has a greater diameter, is shorter and is more vertical than the left. It forms an angle of about 30 degrees with the vertical compared to 43 degree on the left. Its average length is 2.3 cm compared to 5.4 cm on the left. Its average diameter in an adult male is about 17 mm compared to 15 mm on the left. The length of the right principle bronchus is 1.5 cm in infants and 2.0 cm in children, whereas on the left side, these lengths are 2.5 and 3.0 cm respectively.

During inspiration, the carina and the lung roots move forwards and downwards, expanding the diameters of the trachea and bronchi. So it becomes easier to grasp a bronchial FB during inspiration.

In the infant, the chances for respiratory failure are higher, because :

1. The infant has a very low respiratory reserve.
2. The infant and young child have high chances of airway obstruction due to narrow airway and high peripheral airway resistance.
3. His BMR and oxygen consumption per minute are more and heat loss is quite considerable which causes dehydration with rapid rate of respiration.
4. Functional Residual Capacity (FRC) of the lungs is less.
5. When the FB is to be removed, the lumen of the required bronchoscope is very narrow and affords only a narrow, mono-ocular tunnel vision.

Pathogenesis and Clinical Features

Chevalier Jackson (1936)[5] was the first to point out that 90% of the inhaled FBs are a result of carelessness. It is less common for the otorhinolaryngologist to get these patients directly. Most of them are referred to him from pediatric clinics/wards or emergency. A search of literature reveals that virtually anything that can enter the larynx, can be inhaled. But most of the inhaled foreign bodies are nuts and vegetable seeds, small pieces of toys or jewelry, fish bones and whistles. Usually, sharp and linear objects tend to get lodged in the larynx while smaller and smoother, roundish objects enter the trachea/bronchi.

The incidence is the commonest during less than 3 years of age (Table 10.1). Infants and toddlers tend to put things into their mouths haphazardly and if it happens while they are playing, laughing, crying or are just being careless (their gag and cough reflexes not being the best at this age and juncture), they tend to inhale the object. Many times, this event is not witnessed (Table 10.2) and the initial choking and coughing that the inhalation triggers, goes unnoticed. Incidentally, croup also occurs at less than 3 years of age. Hence diagnosis may become difficult because of similar clinical features. The time lag between inhalation and diagnosis is very important from the point of view of morbidity and mortality. Unfortunately, this time lag is not always short (Table 10.3).

Expiratory coughing and spasms are defensive devices, which prevent the FB from being sucked into the larynx / trachea / bronchi. However, factors like how long these defenses can

Table 10.1: Age wise distribution of inhaled foreign bodies

Age	*Rothman*[1] *bockman*	*Brown Clerk*[6]	*Cohen et al*[2]	*Shah V.H*[7]
0-1 yr	39	11	19	189
1-2 yrs	93	46	63	347
2-3 yrs	442	22	23	208
3-4 yrs	12	2	9	86
4-5 yrs	11	2	3	45
5-6 yrs	5	3	4	44
6-7 yrs	6	2	8	19
7-12 yrs	17	13	14	45

Table 10.2: History of aspiration

History of Aspiration	*Shah V.H*[7]	*Rothman becknan*[1]	*Kim et al*[8]
Spontaneously given	32%	85%	85%
On interrogation	44%	13%	14%
No history of Aspiration	24%	2%	1%

Table 10.3: Time taken between aspiration and diagnosis

Days	*Kim et al*[8]	*Cohen et al*[2]	*Strome*[10]	*Shah V.H*[7]
0-1	45%	42%	34%	17%
2-7	23%	20%	12%	33%
8-15	15%	22%	12%	22%
16-30	17%	0%	12%	15%
Over 30 days	0%	16%	30%	13%

hold, the sharpness of edges of the FB, coincidence of occurrence of spasm, the alignment of FB in the glottis at that point of time and its size vis-à-vis the lumen, determine whether the object will get thrown out or impacted. Even a forceful cough fails to expel a FB with sharp projections or if it is caught securely in the subglottis or bronchial walls. Sometimes, a positive history of coughing out a FB may be available but unless the patient returns to normalcy, alertness will still be required to check for any residual or extra FB in the air passage.

If the shape and size of the FB is such that it cannot cross the glottic aperture, it settles there. Glottic FBs, obviously, lie in the sagittal plane. A FB in larynx causes bouts of choking, coughing, hoarse cries, restlessness and dyspnoea. The child gets stridulous and exhausted from breathing against resistance. Chest movements are pronounced but bilaterally symmetrical. Air entry in both lungs is equal, though reduced and there are conducted sounds. There is tachypnoea and tachycardia, which may worsen to cyanosis. In case the FB is big and obliterating the lumen, but can flutter with respiration, this allows some air passage for survival. The FB reaction can extend to the surroundings, causing increased salivation, gurgling sounds and refusal to take solid feeds.

This state of affairs, in the absence of a positive witness of aspiration of FB, can be misdiagnosed as acute laryngitis or acute laryngotracheobronchitis.

Children quiten down after an initial phase of coughing and choking because of the fatigue of cough reflex, perhaps due to adaptation of surface sensory receptors to the presence of foreign body. This sets in a type of chronic phase. The parents feel that the child is better and do not take him to the hospital. However, when the child continues to have cough and if fever also intervenes, the baby is taken to a doctor.

Those FBs, which cross the larynx but fail to enter the bronchial lumen, remain in the trachea and usually flutter with respiration. They get impacted if they are sharp edged. If they are smooth walled, they settle at the carina and may shift from side to side, blocking one or the other bronchus, producing shifting signs in the lungs.

More than 80 per cent of FBs have a smooth passage into one of the bronchi (Table 10.4). There is some controversy about the chosen bronchus, with a suggestion (Ghosh, 1999),[11] that in children below the age of 5, the FB is more likely to be aspirated in to the left bronchus while it is the right one in the older ones. However, a further search of literature[12] reveals that majority of studies find the FB lodging more in the right bronchus (Table 10.5). In small children, the

Table 10.4: Site of lodging of inhaled foreign bodies

Site	*Pyman C.*[9]	*Kim et al*[8]	*Cohen et al*[2]	*Shah V.H.*[7]	*Brown and clerk*[6]
Laryngeal	8.7%	0%	0%	0.03%	0%
Tracheal	5.7%	7%	9%	7%	4%
Bronchial	85.6%	86%	82%	84.97%	84%
Not found	0%	7%	9%	8%	12%

Table 10.5: Details of lodging of foreign bodies

Site	*Kim et al*[8]	*Brown and Clerk*[6]	*Cohen et al*[2]	*Shah V.H*[7]
Right bronchus	50%	48%	39%	47%
Left bronchus	30%	36%	43%	31%
Right lower lobe	2%	0%	0%	3%
Left lower lobe	4%	0%	0%	4%
Trachea	7%	12%	9%	7%
Glottis	0%	0%	0%	0.03%
Not found	7%	12%	9%	8%

septum at the carina is less pronounced. So there is an even chance of an inhaled object going to either side. However, with increasing age, the right bronchus gets straighter in alignment with trachea than the left and is also slightly wider. So it receives more inhaled objects than left.

A FB with a hollow lumen like a whistle causes less trouble unless the lumen is clogged with thick secretions or crusts. It can even be diagnosed by loud whistling sounds – a whistle effect in the tracheobronchial lumen itself. On the other hand, sharp FBs produce local trauma and edema. Vegetable FBs, like peanuts, are quite common and they are worse off because being small, they tend to go deep in to bronchus. Once impacted, they trigger inflammatory reaction due to their lipoid content. Such a FB blocks air entry to a segment leading to collapse consolidation. If on the other hand, a FB acts as a valve, allowing air in with each inspiration but getting blocked on expiration, it produces emphysema. Sooner or later, infection sets in leading to typical signs of reduced air entry to one side and rhonchi and crepitations at a localized area with or without tubular breathing (Tables 10.6 and 10.7). The signs of pneumonitis can appear

Table 10.6: Symptoms in cases of foreign body bronchus

Symptom	*Kim et al*[8]	*Rothman and becknan*[1]	*Shah V.H*[7]
Cough	59%	58%	60%
Wheezing	57%	54%	52%
Respiratory distress	22%	20%	32%
Fever	24%	27%	28%
No history of Aspiration	5%	0%	2%

Table 10.7: Signs in cases of bronchial foreign bodies

Sign	*Kim et al*[8]	*Shah V.H.*[7]
Diminished air entry on one	66%	72%
Cyanosis	5%	1%
Wheezing	38%	48%
Rhonchi	37%	38%
Stridor	13%	8%
Rales	2%	7%

as early as in 24 hrs. The infection may lead to abscess formation. Children presenting with solitary lung abscess, lung collapse and bronchiectasis must be suspected for inhaled FBs.

FBs with long history present with recurrent lung infections, intractable cough and atypical asthma.

Radiological Findings (Table 10.8)

A plane X-ray chest in AP during inspiration and expiration and lateral views including the neck are necessary both for documentation as well as to the pulmonary status and site of obstruction. Radiologically opaque FBs are more common in the esophagus and it is usually advisable to repeat the X-ray before the endoscopy to know the exact site of lodgment.

Table 10.8: Radiological findings in bronchial foreign bodies

Finding	*Kim et. al.*[8]	*Rothman beckman*[1]	*Shah V.H*[7]
Obstructive emphysema	37%	60%	55%
Collapse	12%	0%	12%
Consolidation	20%	12%	12%
Radio-opaque foreign body	13%	13%	3%
Lower lobe collapse	6%	8%	6%
Normal X ray	11%	7%	11%

Plane X-ray chest in cases of a tracheobronchial FB in the first 24 hrs is likely to be normal in most cases. In such cases, screening of the chest is more helpful as it will show the mediastinal swing.

The commonest radiological finding in most cases is obstructive emphysema on one side, collapse of the lower lobe on either side. Collapse and/or consolidation of the lung are also diagnostic findings of bronchial obstruction. One case had pneumothorax on one side following violent cough after FB ingestion and another child, a known asthmatic, had surgical emphysema in the neck following FB ingestion. Total collapse of the lung on either side is also seen in cases where bronchial obstruction is total, as in the case of a swollen vegetative FB. Changing consolidation on either side is almost diagnostic of a shifting FB.

There can be different types of bronchial obstructions, related to FB aspiration. The bypass valve partially obstructs in both phases of respiration. Aeration beyond obstruction occurs, although at a diminished rate, so the chest X-ray is normal. As many as 20% of children with bronchial FBs and more than half of those with tracheal FBs show no radiographic abnormality. Small, flat or oblong organic FBs, such as watermelon or sunflower seeds, often produce no abnormality in chest film.

The check valve obstruction, in which air can be inhaled but cannot pass during exhalation, produces obstructive emphysema on the involved side. Both inspiratory and expiratory radiographs are required to make this diagnosis. Mediastinal shift will occur towards the normal side.

If the FB becomes impacted on inspiration, yet dislodges on expiration, a ball valve obstruction results. This happens with a smooth round FB like a whole peanut. This leads to early atelectasis and collapse with mediastinal shift towards the involved side.

Finally complete blockage by a large FB produces a stop valve obstruction. Air passage is prevented on both inhalation and exhalation. This results in consolidation of the involved segment with subsequent collapse.

Any of these types of obstructions can lead to pneumonia.

Although radiographic signs are helpful in reaching the diagnosis when supported by a history of aspiration and clinical signs, these findings are not pathognomonic and carry a sensitivity of 68 per cent when compared to bronchoscopic findings.

Computerized Tomography (CT) is an excellent method to study the cross-sectional pathology of trachea while MRI is useful for delineation of vascular abnormalities and masses compressing the airway.

Strategies for Removal

Instruments and Equipment

For direct laryngoscopy, Storz slotted or Jackson pediatric laryngoscopes are used. Phillips straight blade, anesthetist's laryngoscope is handy for a child.

Fibreoptic conventional rigid endoscopes with halogen light source (cold light fountain with 250 watts halogen lamp and built in spare bulbs) with two outlets and increasing steps of brightness are the basic requirements along with various types of FB holding forceps. Storz ventilating bronchoscopes from size 2.5 mm to 6.0 mm with distal fibreoptic illumination are used. One must remember that the size 2.5 to 6.0 mm means the inner (and not the outer) diameter. Guide to use the correct size of bronchoscope according to the age of the child is given in Table 10.9 below.

Table 10.9: Guide to use the correct size of bronchoscope according to the age of the child

Age	*Size*	*True external diameter*
Neonate	2.5mm	4.0mm
Infant	3.0mm	5.0mm
Six months to one and a half years	3.5mm	5.7mm
Two to three years	4.0mm	7.0mm
Three and a half to eight years	5.0mm	7.8mm
Over eight years	6.0mm	8.2mm

Various types of foreign body holding forceps, suction cannulas and suction tube are required.

0 degree and 30 degrees Hopkins Telescopes, with xenon light source, are used for diagnostic and photographic purposes.

Flexible fibreoptic laryngoscope and pediatric bronchoscope are ideal for diagnostic purposes and are not useful for any endoscopic surgical procedure in an infant or child. Advantages of rigid endoscopes are manifold. They not only provide superb illumination, natural color production, wide angle viewing but also allow instrumentation for suction, FB removal, collection of aspiration samples and biopsy (Table 10.10).

Operating Room Setup

Besides having the above-mentioned instruments and equipment, we need to have a proper operating room layout.

The surgeon sits at the head end while the anesthetist stands on the patient's left side. Constant monitoring of heart and oxygen level is a must. Cardiopulmonary monitor and pulse oxymeter should be kept over the anesthetist's trolley so that the anesthetist can easily see them.

Table 10.10: General advantages and disadvantages of rigid and flexible endoscopy

Rigid endoscopy		*Flexible endoscopy*	
Advantages	*Disadvantages*	*Advantages*	*Disadvantages*
1. It functions as a protected airway for oxygenation and anesthesia.	1. Inability to reach the distal airway.	1. Very useful in nursery and pediatric ICU as it can be passed through endotracheal tube.	1. It compromises an already obstructed airway.
2. Offers opportunity to treat lesions.	2. Cannot be used under local anesthesia.	2. Does not require general anesthesia.	2. Does not allow instrumentation.
3. Much safer for FB removal.	3. More risky and traumatic.	3. Allows study of physiological and functional assessment of pediatric airway and dynamics of supraglottic structures, larynx and trachea.	3. Not suitable for removal of foreign bodies, benign lesions and thick secretions.
4. Allows use of multiple instruments and telescopes.	4. Contraindicated in cases of cervical disorders and coagulopathies.	4. Less risky and less traumatic.	4. 2.7 mm bronchoscope does not have suction channel.
5. Easier removal of granulation tissue, thick secretions and hardened fibrin plugs.		5. Useful in postoperative assessment in cases where surgery has been done for pediatric airway.	5. Does not allow use of CO_2 laser.
6. Allows use of CO2 laser.		6. Useful for proper segmental bronchogram before lung surgery.	
		7. Useful for aspiration of secretions for culture and sensitivity test.	
		8. Can be used safely in cases of immunocompromised patients, pulmonary infiltrates of carcinoma, cervical spine disorders and in coagulopathies.	
		9. More safe and has less complications.	
		10. Avoids more expensive diagnostic tools like CT scan, barium swallow and fluoroscopy.	

The light source is kept behind the right hand side of the surgeon, the instrument trolley is also to his right and the assistant nurse should stand on the patient's right side. Suction operates from the left, as it is convenient both to the anesthetist and the surgeon. A separate instrument trolley and tracheostomy set is always kept ready on the side. The photographic equipment with the xenon light source is also placed on the right side.

Before taking the child for endoscopy, the surgeon, anesthetist and assistant nurse should check all the equipments and run them. It is always better to have an extra light source and suction machine ready in case of failure. At places, where power failures are frequent, an electronic generator must be kept ready, which can provide enough electric power to run the light source, monitors and suction machines. Extra oxygen and gas cylinders should also be kept ready with all emergency drugs and all sizes of endotracheal tubes. Few minutes spent on a preliminary check up on the working of all necessary and vital equipments can prevent many complications and is often life saving.

Ideal anesthesia for a child undergoing endoscopic procedure, where airway is partially obstructed, demands the need of an experienced and senior anesthetist, ably assisted by equally experienced assistants. In most cases, the success of the procedure is more due to the vigilant anesthetist who takes full charge of the situation and oxygenates the child adequately. With slight evidence of bradycardia or fall in oxygen level, the endoscopist should move out and give all space and assistance to the anesthetist so as to avoid cardiac arrest. The surgeon should be present when the patient is being anesthetized because the patient may have airway obstruction before and during induction of anesthesia.

The basic requirements of ideal anesthesia are simple rapid induction, prompt functional recovery, immobile unobstructed larynx, no time restriction and minimal aspiration and secretions. Oxygenation is maintained with jet ventilation and constant monitoring of cardiopulmonary functions. Many endoscopists prefer induction with inhalation anesthesia or using halothane and maintain spontaneous breathing throughout the procedure, so as to maintain the dynamic movement of the tracheobronchial tree. Some use I.V. ketamine instead of Pentothal, but it is not safe in endoscopy procedure, as it does not abolish the pharyngeal and laryngeal reflex. Topical spray of 4% Xylocaine is very useful as it virtually abolishes laryngeal spasm and vagus reflex.

Before starting the anesthesia, a firm I.V. line should be established with a scalp vein cannula or intracath and infusion should be started. In case of a small chubby child, it is always difficult to get the vein once it is lost and especially when it is needed most, when the child develops bradycardia or cardiac arrest. The success of FB removal from respiratory tract largely depends on the anesthesia and hence all precautions should be taken for its safety.

Technique of Endoscopic Removal

At any given time, endoscopy procedure demands gentleness on the part of the surgeon. No force should be used during the introduction and it should be done under constant vision. It should be swift and atraumatic. The surgeon has to be assisted by an experienced nurse who is not only acquainted with his movements and gestures but can predict what may be going on in his mind and also can anticipate which forceps, suction cannula or other instruments he will need during the procedure. Proper assistance and anticipation goes a long way in a successful surgery. It is teamwork between the surgeon, anesthetist and assisting nurse and hence it requires proper understanding of each other's technique and temperament during the procedure.

Foreign Body in the Larynx

A foreign body in the larynx usually lodges in subglottic region or in the supraglottic region but seldom in glottis. It may be safer to do a tracheostomy before removing the same. The child is placed on the table so that the head is at the superior margin of the table. Direct laryngoscopy is done after the child is put under anesthesia with open mask method and spontaneous breathing. After removal of open mask, the larynx should be sprayed with 4% Xylocaine. An adequate size of hand held laryngoscope with straight blade should be introduced. A saline soaked gauze sponge is placed over the upper gum to protect the upper teeth. Care should be taken to avoid trauma to the lips, oral cavity, the fauces and the pharynx during the introduction of the laryngoscope. The child's neck should be gently extended so as to visualize the epiglottis and then it should be lifted gently to examine the rest of the larynx. Sometimes light pressure is required externally over the larynx for better visualization. The FB is seen and is gently extricated, causing minimal damage to the tissues, if at all.

Precautions During Laryngoscopy

The commonest complication that can occur during direct laryngoscopy in a child is subglottic edema following trauma to the larynx. This can be carefully avoided by gentle handling and care during instrumentation. Other safety factors that must be considered are maintenance of hydration and full suction of secretions and blood during and after the procedure. It is very essential to see the complete return of muscular tone, cough reflex, cry and whether they can support their own airway or not.

In rare instances (Kamath *et al*, 1999),[14] when a FB is impacted in subglottis, a laryngofissure approach may be needed.

Tracheobronchial Foreign Bodies

As a general rule, the otolaryngologist must proceed with endoscopic intervention as soon as there is a suspicion of presence of a tracheobroncheal FB. Although the procedure is to be done as soon as possible, the surgeon should not rush in to it without a careful and meticulous preparation. It is a tenuous procedure. Hypoxia or anoxia can occur any time and hence all equipments must be carefully chosen, assembled and be ready for use before administration of anesthetic agent. The surgeon and the anesthetist should be prepared to assure immediate control of the airway.

Holinger[13] has very rightly said, "If two hours are spent in preparations, the safe endoscopic procedure may take two minutes. But if only two minutes are taken for preparation, the endoscopist may find himself attempting makeshift ineffective procedure for next two hours."

Anesthesia

There are two good alternatives:

i. Inhalation anesthesia with spontaneous breathing (halothane, nitrous oxide, oxygen).
ii. Induction with sodium pentothal, relaxation with scoline, oxygenation with face mask, spraying the larynx with 4% Xylocaine, again oxygenation with face mask to be followed by introduction of bronchoscope and maintenance of oxygenation with jet ventilation, with repeat dose of scoline if necessary. The total relaxation makes tracheobronchial tree completely open and it is easier to visualize and catch the FB.

The anesthetist after discussing with the surgeon chooses the right method depending on the demands of that particular case.

Technique of Removal

Rigid ventilating fibreoptic bronchoscope with telescopic visualization is the instrument of choice. This allows direct access to airway, excellent visualization, continuous administration of oxygen and anesthetic agents and suitable conduit for the introduction and extraction of forceps and suction tube. A bronchoscope of appropriate dimension for the patient is selected. A smaller diameter bronchoscope should always be kept ready for use in the event of an unsuspected airway narrowing. The selected bronchoscope should be checked for proper illumination and through and through vision. Sometimes an old clot lying near the distal part of the fibreoptic carrier may diminish the intensity of light as well as obstruct vision. Endoscopes should always be cleaned properly before and after their use. A correct size of suction cannula should be checked for the patency of its lumen and ability to pass through the bronchoscope.

The selection of extraction forceps is determined by the nature of suspected FB. During a determined history taking, most of the parents will be able to identify the nature of FB and if possible, may also be able to produce its replica. In most cases, the FB is vegetative and usually a peanut. A variety of forceps, like crocodile, alligator, toothed, non- toothed, serrated, flat, cupped, peanut (both angled and straight), are available. The forceps should be such that it assures a firm grip of the FB and does not damage the bronchial mucosa. It should also have a firm and straight shaft so that it does not wobble or obscure the view when it is put to work.

It is always better to first view the child's larynx with the Phillips straight bladed laryngoscope, which will help in lifting the epiglottis. It should be held in the left hand, with proper care as already explained. Bronchoscope should then be held in right hand with pen hold grip and should be gently glided in to the glottis with its tip upwards and underneath the epiglottis. Then loosen the grip over the laryngoscope, which will allow you to observe the vocal cords through the bronchoscope. Then gently slip the endoscope into the trachea. If the neck had earlier to be extended, release it slowly to see the whole lumen of the trachea. Then gently rotate the tip of the bronchoscope by 90 degree so that you can hold the handle of the bronchoscope properly. The anesthetist then starts inflating the lungs with jet ventilation by the side of the bronchoscope.

Sometimes the bronchoscope may slips into esophagus instead of entering the trachea. Failure to identify the patent lumen with tracheal rings and inability to inflate the lungs with jet ventilation should alert the endoscopist that he is not in the air passage.

Once you are convinced that the bronchoscope is in the trachea, then glide it over the thumb of your left hand, which is holding the upper jaw of the child. Never use undue force and glide the endoscope under vision. Carina is then identified. It is easy to introduce the bronchoscope into the right main bronchus with slight angulation towards the left. It can then be withdrawn slightly and angled to the right so as to visualize the left main bronchus. Suction should be used from time to time to clear the secretions, which may obstruct the view.

Loose FBs in trachea can be a tricky affair. Do not try to catch them when they are free in trachea. Try to push them down and let them lodge over the carina or at the entrance of the right bronchus. Then it is easier to catch them and remove. Such FBs should be removed at the earliest as they may get stuck in subglottic region and can cause total airway obstruction.

Removal of FB from the bronchus is a matter of skill and art and it has to be mastered with experience. Once the FB is located in a bronchus, adequate suction should be done to identify the type of the FB. Sometimes in a case of chronic bronchial obstruction of long duration, the bronchus is full of purulent secretions and granulation tissues around the old FB.

The bronchoscope should be aligned with the bronchus and the FB in one straight line. The FB forceps with closed blades should then be introduced and the blades are opened after it crosses the tip of bronchoscope and then the FB should be caught firmly and brought near the tip of the bronchoscope with gentle but firm withdrawal of forceps. Then the forceps and the bronchoscope should be gently withdrawn in one assembly till it reaches the glottis. At this juncture, care should be taken not to lose the FB as it invariably gets caught in the anterior part of the glottis. The bronchoscope should be tilted slightly upwards so that its tip with held FB passes out through the posterior part of the glottis, which is wider and spacious. If it is realized that the FB cannot come out of the trachea for whatever reasons, it should be retuned to the carina and a quick decision should be taken to do a tracheostomy and deliver the FB through the tracheostome.

After the removal of FB, the anesthetist should oxygenate the patient with open mask and then allow the surgeon to reintroduce the bronchoscope to inspect the tracheobronchial tree for the possibility of remnants or rarely, a second FB. The tracheobronchial tree should then be cleaned properly with suction and the bronchoscope is kept in trachea for proper oxygenation till the child comes out of the effect of the relaxant and starts breathing spontaneously. The bronchoscope is then withdrawn and anesthetist oxygenates the breathing child. Alternatively, the anesthetist may opt to intubate the child at this stage and lead him through a smooth recovery. The anesthetist and the surgeon should not leave the child till its muscle tone returns to normal, cough reflex is present and the child starts crying. Air entry is checked on either side, the head end of the table is then lowered and the child is kept in a left lateral position before shifting to the wards.

If, following this surgery, there is evidence of subglottic edema by way of brassy cough or stridor, the child is given I.V. steroids and observed.

Complications

Intraoperative

1. Problems due to defective, inadequate and improper equipments.
2. Hypoxia, hypercarbia, respiratory acidosis, cardiac arrhythmia, bradycardia, cardiac arrest. Proper atropinization before every dose of relaxant may prevent cardiac arrythmia.
3. Laryngeal or subglottic edema due to oversized endoscopes and repeated instrumentation.
4. Loss of I.V. line. Preferably use intracath right at the beginning with I.V. drip.
5. Subglottic impaction of a FB while removal through the glottis. This would impair ventilation and FB has to be pushed down to one of the main bronchi.

Postoperative

1. *Laryngospasm* This can be avoided by spraying of the larynx with 4% xylocaine and not removing the endoscope till the child starts breathing on its own and cough reflex has returned.
2. *Laryngeal edema* This can be avoided by gentle instrumentation and can be treated in time with I.V. steroids.
3. *Aspiration of secretions or vomitus* This can be prevented by proper suction of the throat before sending the child to the wards. One must wait till its muscular tone and reflexes have regained fully.
4. A postoperative chest X-ray is mandatory and if it reveals pneumothorax, a chest surgeon should be called to put in a chest tube.

It should be remembered that a sharp metallic FB while being inhaled, could itself cause some rupture and leakage of air, leading to conditions like surgical emphysema, mediastinal emphysema or pneumothorax (Fig. 10.1).

Pneumonitis and lung abscess may also occur postoperatively and should be dealt with in collaboration with the chest physician and chest surgeon.

Immediate care should be taken to treat these complications, as they all can be fatal.

Some Representative Case Reports

Of the numerous inhaled FBs removed by the authors, few, chosen for their representative nature are summarily being given here.

1. R.Y., a one year old male child presented with a history of inhalation of a piece of silver jewelry (Jhumka, with sharp edges, a week before his admission on 9th August, 1993. The child had violent cough, mild fever, inspiratory stridor, conducted sounds, reduced air entry to right side, bilateral rhonchi and scattered crepitations. His HbSaO2 on room air was 90%. Chest X ray revealed a metallic FB hanging from carina into the right bronchus, with surgical emphysema, mediastinal emphysema and features of air trapping (Fig. 10.1). Bronchoscopic removal of the FB presented no difficulties and the child quickly recovered, having been put on ampicillin and steroids postoperatively. This case was significant since there were features of air leak into mediastinum and neck spaces caused by the FB itself due to its sharp cutting edges, worsened by violent coughing.
2. N., a 10 months old male child, presented on 10th June, 1992 with a history of inhaling a gram seed 9 days earlier. The infant had a hacking type of cough and reduced air entry to left lung. An X ray chest showed obstructive emphysema on the left side with shift of heart and mediastinum to the right (Fig. 10.2). However, while a surgery was being planned, the

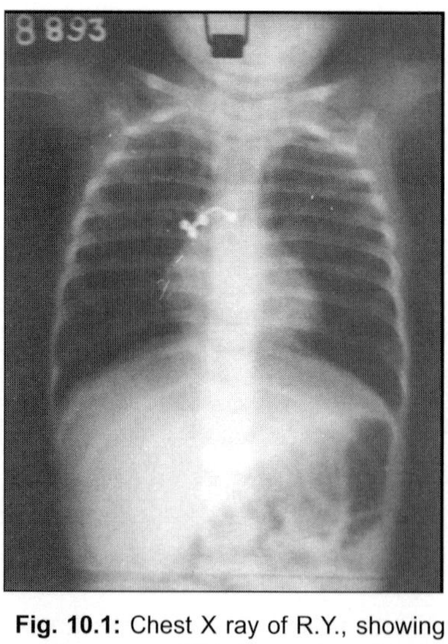

Fig. 10.1: Chest X ray of R.Y., showing a radio-opaque FB in the region of carina and right main bronchus with surgical emphysema and features of air trapping. Heart shadow appears normal.

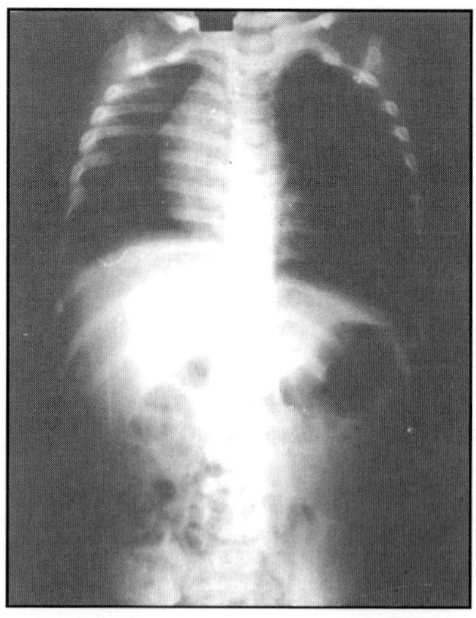

Fig. 10.2: Chest X ray of N. There is obstructive emphysema in the left lung with shift of heart and mediastinum to the right.

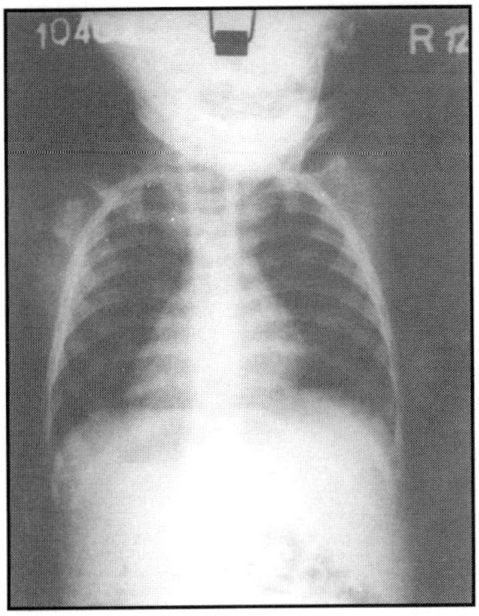

Fig. 10.3: Normal chest x ray of N, after the FB was coughed out.

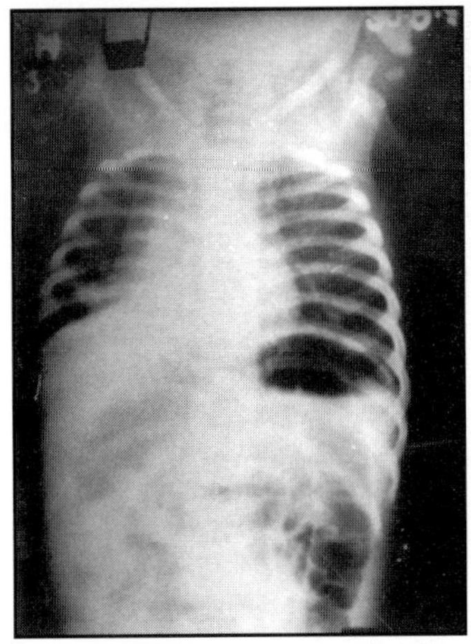

Fig. 10.4: X ray chest of S.D. Features of tracheal shift to the right with collapse-consolidation in the upper and mid-zone right lung. Heart and mediastinum are shifted to the right. Left lung shows redistribution of flow with compensatory emphysema of right lower lobe.

child coughed out the gram seed and the lung turned normal (Fig. 10.3). No treatment needed to be given.

3. S.D., a 6 months old male child, presented on 30th May, 1994, with a history of having choked, with violent cough and bad respiration while ingesting some food items. There was a previous history of cough and cold and the infant had received treatment for bronchopneumonia two months back. On examination, the infant was found irritable, febrile, had distressed breathing with two-way stridor. On auscultation, the chest revealed adventitious sounds. Air entry was reduced on right. An X ray chest (Fig. 10.4) showed tracheal shift to the right, collapse consolidation in upper and mid zones in the right lung, heart and mediastinal shift to the right and compensatory emphysema in the lower lobe right side. Left lung showed redistribution of flow. An unsuccessful attempt at bronchoscopic removal by another colleague saw the condition turning in to a total right lung collapse (Fig. 10.5). A repeat bronchoscopy was done immediately and a "ber" seed was extracted from the right main bronchus. Respiration immediately became normal and a check X-ray showed normalcy (Fig. 10.6).
4. G.S.S., 68 years male, a case of chronic bronchial asthma, presented at the emergency with an acute attack on 16th January, 1999. Having been given treatment there, he decided to have a very loose tooth removed in dental clinic. The tooth was extracted but it somehow slipped and got inhaled into the right bronchus (Fig. 10.7). The patient had no particular symptoms because of this incidence apart from some cough. Bronchoscopic removal done the same afternoon presented no problems.

Few things are evident from these case studies. Infants and small children, because of the small size of their bronchial lumen, tend to have quick lung collapse. But when the offending FBs are neatly removed, return to normalcy quickly. In adults, an inhaled FB usually does not cause grave symptoms.

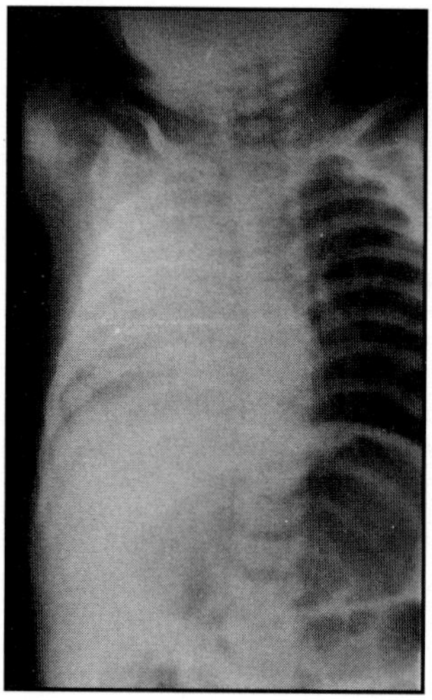

Fig. 10.5: X ray chest showing total collapse of right lung, opaque right hemithorax with shift of heart and mediastinum to the right.

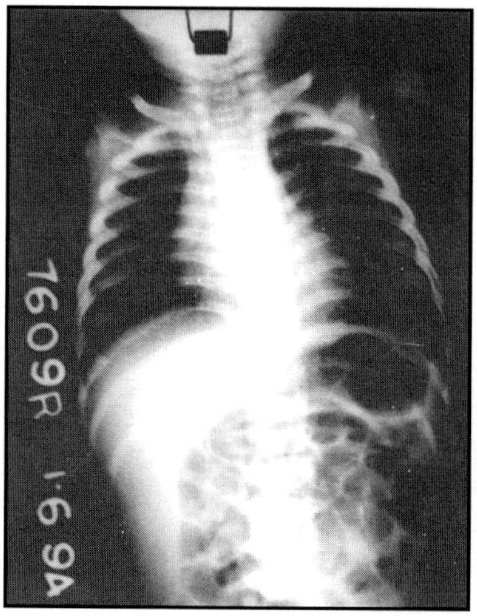

Fig. 10.6: Postoperative normal X ray chest of the same child.

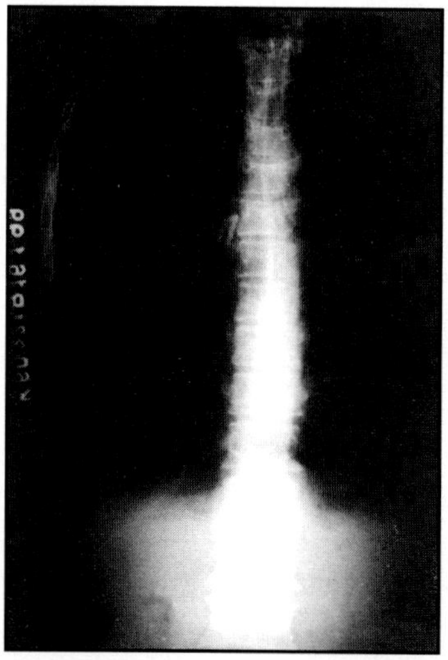

Fig. 10.7: X ray chest of G.S.S. Chronic obstructive pulmonary disease with a tooth (FB) in the right main bronchus.

An inhaled FB is a challenging situation both for the ENT surgeon and the anesthetist. Its removal requires skill, planning, presence of mind and quick decision-making.

REFERENCES

1. Rothman BF, Boeckman CR. Foreign bodies in the larynx and tracheobronchial tree in children. A review of 225 cases. Ann Otol Rhinol Laryngol 1980; 89:434-36.
2. Cohen SR, Herbert WI, Lewis GB, Geller KA. Foreign bodies in the airway. Five year retrospective study with special reference to management. Ann Otol Rhinol Laryngol 1980; 89:437-42.

3. Ward PH, Berci G, Calcaterra TC. Advances in endoscopic examination of the respiratory system. Ann Rhinol. Laryngol. 1974; 83:7654-60.
4. Hopkins HH. Endoscopy. Appleton Century Crofts, New York, 1976; pp.17.
5. Jackson C and Jackson CL. Quoted by Holinger P.H. and Holinger C.D. (1978). Use of open tube bronchoscope in the extraction of foreign bodies. Chest 1936; 73:721-26.
6. Brown DA and Clark CM. Inhaled foreign bodies in children. Med. J. Australia 1983; 2:322-26.
7. Shah VH. Pediatric endoscopy. Published by V.H. Shah, on behalf of Sheth P.T. Surat General hospital, Surat, India, 1997.
8. Kim IG, Bremmit WM, Humphrey A. Foreign body in the airway : a review of 202 cases. Laryngoscope 1973; 83:347-54.
9. Pyman C. Inhaled foreign bodies in childhood – a review of 230 cases. Med. J. Australia 1971; 1:62-68.
10. Strome M. Tracheobronchial foreign bodies : an updated approach. Ann Otol Rhinol Laryngol 1977; 86:649-54.
11. Ghosh P. Foreign bodies in ear, nose and throat (predictions and management). Indian J Otolaryngol and HNS surgery. August 1999: 2-5
12. Swenson G. Foreign bodies in the tracheobroncheal tree. Special reference to experience in 97 children. Int J Ped Otorhinolaryngo 1985; l.61:5-17.
13. Holinger LD. Etiology of stridor in the neonate, infant and child. Ann Otol Rhinol Laryngol. 1980; 89:397-400.
14. Kamath MP, Murthy PS, Hazarika P. A case of foreign body in the subglottic region. Indian J Otolaryngol and HNS surgery 1999:6-8.

Index

T

U

V

W

X

READER SUGGESTIONS SHEET

Please help us to improve the quality of our publications by completing and returning this sheet to us.

Author/Title: **Challenges in Otorhinolaryngology *By Anil Malhotra, Milind Kirtane***

Your name and address:

Phone and Fax:

e-mail address:

How did you hear about this book? [please tick appropriate box (es)]

- ☐ Direct mail from publisher
- ☐ Conference
- ☐ Bookshop
- ☐ Book review
- ☐ Lecturer recommendation
- ☐ Friends
- ☐ Other (please specify)
- ☐ Website

Type of purchase: ☐ Direct purchase ☐ Bookshop ☐ Friends

Do you have any brief comments on the book?

Please return this sheet to the name and address given below.

JAYPEE BROTHERS
MEDICAL PUBLISHERS (P) LTD
EMCA House, 23/23B Ansari Road, Daryaganj
New Delhi 110 002, India